Different Baby, Different Story

Different Baby, Different Story

Pregnancy and Parenting after Loss

JOANN O'LEARY, LYNNDA PARKER,
MARGARET M. MURPHY, AND JANE WARLAND

ROWMAN & LITTLEFIELD
Lanham • Boulder • New York • London

Published by Rowman & Littlefield
An imprint of The Rowman & Littlefield Publishing Group, Inc.
4501 Forbes Boulevard, Suite 200, Lanham, Maryland 20706
www.rowman.com

6 Tinworth Street, London SE11 5AL, United Kingdom

British Library Cataloguing in Publication Information Available

Library of Congress Cataloging-in-Publication Data

Names: O'Leary, Joann, author. | Parker, Lynnda, 1951– author. | Murphy,
   Margaret M., 1967– author. | Warland, Jane, 1957– author.
Title: Different baby, different story : pregnancy and parenting after loss
   / Joann O'Leary, Lynnda Parker, Margaret M. Murphy, and Jane Warland.
Description: Lanham : Rowman & Littlefield, [2020] | Includes
   bibliographical references and index. | Summary: "Through the words of
   parents, siblings, and family members this book assists readers through
   the complex journey of a pregnancy following loss. With practical advice
   on self-advocacy, expectant parents gain insights to help them to work
   with health care professionals, mental health professionals, and their
   own families, friends and coworkers"— Provided by publisher.
Identifiers: LCCN 2020036219 (print) | LCCN 2020036220 (ebook) | ISBN
   9781538125328 (cloth) | ISBN 9781538125335 (epub)
Subjects: LCSH: Subsequent pregnancy—Psychological aspects. |
   Childbirth—Psychological aspects. | Fetal death. | Perinatal death. |
   Parental grief. | Parenting—Psychological aspects.
Classification: LCC RG560 .O44 2020 (print) | LCC RG560 (ebook) | DDC
   618.2—dc23
LC record available at https://lccn.loc.gov/2020036219
LC ebook record available at https://lccn.loc.gov/2020036220

Contents

Acknowledgments

This book contains all four authors' combined research and years of clinical practice with families pregnant after the loss of a baby. It incorporates major revisions of previous books and chapters written by the authors and material from videos produced by Dr. O'Leary and Ms. Parker. Special thanks to the Bush Foundation in St. Paul, Minnesota, which funded Dr. O'Leary's original research. Dr. Warland also brings the perspective of a bereaved parent to this work in honor of her deceased baby Emma and her "rainbow" baby Sarah. Dr. Murphy would like to thank her doctoral research supervisors; special thanks to her husband Tony, her constant support and sounding board, and she dedicates this book to her children, Luke, Lily, and Izzy, who remain her greatest achievement. We are all grateful for the support given by our families, who endured us during the months this book was in production. Most of all, this book could not have been written without the many families who have shared their stories with us, for which we are all grateful.

Additional thanks go to:

Darrell Peterson, bereaved father to Elize, for reviewing the fathers chapter

Lynn Stylianou Jensen, bereaved grandmother to Hansel, Carolyne, Lillian, and Frank, for reviewing chapter 13: "The Ripple Effect"

Amanda Feltmann for sharing her letter to family and friends of expectations before her rainbow daughter Corel's birth following the loss of Juniper

Sid and Christine Chang for sharing their letter on moving forward with their sons and missing Madison

Diana Le-Cabrera for her mantra signs

Lisa Paraku, in New Zealand, for permission to use her words in the chapters "Beautiful Chaos," "Uncomfortable Truths," and "Beautiful Babies Breathing"

Anna Calix, in memory of Liam: labor picture of subsequent birth

Danielle Ondarza, in memory of Jude: postpartum picture

Brittany Day, in memory of Ruby and Sophia: picture of big sister Eliza

Michaela Backiel: birth announcement of her three children, in memory of Jonathan

Mona McNeely: poem in memory of Kevin

Anne Deane: poem in memory of Baily

Keri Padin: Wall of Hope in memory of her deceased children

Dr. Jolene Pearson: flex hold

Suzanne I. Staszak-Silva, executive editor, Rowman & Littlefield, for her support and insight

1

Finding Hope

When the heart is cut or cracked or broken do not clutch it. Let the wound lie open. Let the wind from the good old sea blow in to bathe the wound with salt and let it sting. Let a stray dog lick it. Let a bird fly in the hole and sing a simple song like a tiny bell and let it ring.[1]

This chapter begins your journey from loss to hope, in anticipation of trying again for a new baby, one who will be a sibling to your much-loved, deceased baby.

When the very worst thing imaginable has happened, how can you possibly make any meaning of your baby's death? Pregnancy loss is an event that humans struggle to make sense of. It is not the natural order of things that children should die before their parents, and when that death occurs before birth, your faith in any natural order may be shaken to its core.

HOPE

You are thinking about trying to get pregnant again. What does that mean for you? As humans, we are inherently hopeful beings. In this pregnancy you will be hopeful of a live birth, a positive outcome. Finding hope may be challenging, but the fact that you are looking forward to another pregnancy is, in itself, a hopeful act. Maintaining hope throughout the journey of a pregnancy that follows a loss is an important activity for couples to engage in.

Communication, which may be difficult at times, is key to supporting one another and finding hope. While others may be thinking you did not really know your deceased baby, your identity as a parent and attachment will continue forever. This is normal and to be expected. You are forever changed because of your deceased baby's life and death.

Michael Trout, infant-parent specialist, shares a brief description of his grandmother's story after the loss of her baby in 1920, and who she became as a person because of this loss:[2]

> Maternal (and paternal!) identity changes, following the loss of a baby. I found myself thinking about how confusing it must have been for my grandmother, who was a woman of considerable power, to notice that she wasn't "getting over" the loss of her first daughter as quickly as others expected. She couldn't have articulated, then, that her role as a parent wasn't over when that baby died. She was never the same, but not because she was inadequate at grieving. It would affect her sense of self and her silent fears during subsequent pregnancies.

In your previous pregnancy, particularly if it was your first, you may not have thought of yourself as "really" a parent until your baby came into the outside world. This is probably a reflection of how society views pregnancy. In fact, how often did you hear, "When is your baby due?" They don't understand that your deceased baby made you parents during his or her pregnancy, as you made parenting decisions on his or her behalf every day. The transition to parenthood begins in pregnancy and takes many, many months. Birth itself is only a stepping-stone on the path, not the event itself. As you embark on a new pregnancy, you continue to parent your deceased baby because you are still a parent to that baby.

Society does not fully understand grief. People may be telling you to "get over it" or "move on." Grief does not come without attachment and great love. Often, it comes with complicated feelings of confusion, striving for definition, and a hope that it may ease over time. You loved your baby greatly; therefore you may always feel grief alongside your love for your deceased baby. While time does not make the pain of your loss vanish, it may soften it somewhat.

> You just have to find a good place in your mind and just handle it. See if you can move yourself on from it, you know, and that can make things good for yourself. We weren't forgetting about her. (Iona)

The death of your baby has likely changed you as a person and as a couple. It may have changed your priorities or your outlook on life. Every future experience may be colored by the prism of the loss of your baby. There may be times when you are happy and there may be an element of guilt that goes with that, because you may feel that you are being disloyal to your deceased baby. The journey of pregnancy after loss is one of carrying both hope and grief together.

A question you may ponder if your loss was "only" a miscarriage is: Am I still a parent? You may be surprised that if you google fetal cells, you will learn that cells remain in women's bodies—even babies who die in the first trimester. This may give meaning to why you may still feel the presence of your baby. Regardless of the outcome or gestation of your previous pregnancy, you have been changed as a person, and yes, you are still a mother. The following story, from a book titled *Called to Heal*, illustrates these feelings:[3]

> Healers believe that time is only relative to our physical existence. They explain that when they speak with the ancestors and interact through visions that there is no time. It is as if all things happen simultaneously. We are born; we are alive; we die; we are spirits: it is all happening at the same time. I was taken by surprise when one of the healers told me I had a teenage daughter. I remember thinking: "Aha! I've caught her. She's wrong." But before I had a chance to challenge her, she explained that my daughter was actually the spirit of a baby I had miscarried in the South Pacific. I had never mentioned that I had lived there. I certainly never discussed a miscarriage. Had that child lived she would indeed have been a teenager. In the case of a miscarriage, the healers believe the child will stay with and be raised by the mother. Since there is not time and space in the spirit world, I had been mothering this child all along and would meet her at my death.
>
> This experience that had left vestiges of unresolved grief was brought full circle. At the time the healer told me about my daughter, I saw the child for a moment. She was distant in my peripheral vision, yet I had a strong feel for her personality. I could see she was tall, slender, with long light brown hair. It felt very natural. It was like being with my son after not having seen him for a couple of hours. She was very familiar, as if she lived with me. I could see her smiling. It was very comforting.

Regardless of how your baby died, love endures. As you move forward, your deceased baby continues to be an important member of your family: a baby whom perhaps only you, your partner, or older siblings know. Initially you may grieve for the baby who was, but that may change to grief for the person who was yet to be.

> Honoring her memory and the person she would have been. (Adam)

Below are suggestions other families have offered for honoring their deceased baby that you may find useful. Every family chooses how they might want to do this: honoring your pregnancy and the child that didn't make it through can be healing.

REFLECTIONS

- One mother bought two little booties for her miscarried babies, writing their due dates on the soles. She buried them with the ashes of her father.
- In a paper titled "Affirmation of Our Children Loved and Lifetimes Lost," another mother gave names to her five miscarried children and the dates they would have been born.
- Sometimes when children find out their mother had a miscarriage or a baby whom they did not know about, they help the parents name the baby. After learning about a miscarriage his mother had not talked about, the four-year-old told her, "We should name that baby." The mother now felt her family was complete.
- Another family keeps the memory of their daughter alive by using her name when they are put on a waiting list at a restaurant.
- One woman gave her husband a small potted ivy plant to care for when they lost their first son; she now tends to the plant after eighteen years.
- When a subsequent child was born, the parents gave him their son's name as a middle name.

2

Trying Again

The timeless in you is aware of life's timelessness. And knows that yesterday is but today's memory and tomorrow is today's dream.

—*Kahlil Gibran[1]*

MAKING THE DECISION TO TRY AGAIN

Making the decision to try to get pregnant is one of the biggest decisions you make as a parent. However, for you, the decision is even bigger because now you know babies don't always survive, and you wonder whether to risk trying again. Having lost a child once, pregnancies are never the same again. Can you go through all that pain again?

You might be wondering if:

- You can get pregnant again, or was that the only time?
- You can carry a pregnancy to term, especially if you haven't done so before.
- You can have a healthy baby this time (or at least one who lives).

WHY DID MY BABY DIE?

While searching for a reason why your baby died, it is very common to second-guess decisions you made during your pregnancy. If a definitive reason was not provided, you may always question yourself. But pregnancy loss is more common than most people know and happens for a variety of reasons,

5

and it is rarely linked to a mother's behaviors or actions. In contemplating a future pregnancy, it is important to discuss what happened with your maternity care provider. It will be helpful to understand how your previous loss may impact your next pregnancy. You also may want to discuss any tests you might need before you get pregnant again. If an earlier loss was for genetic reasons, genetic counseling may be in order.

> Before I was pregnant again, I told the doctors how my care would go in the future, what I would need to have different, and asked for their insight on other things. (Amanda)

You also want to learn the medical facts. It may help to know what action is appropriate for you, based on tests, medications, and treatments. For example, if your baby was born preterm, you may want to find out whether there are treatments available that may help prevent this from happening again. If heredity played a part in your situation, you may be referred to a genetic counselor.

> I'm the one that carries a gene that basically could fifty-fifty or 100 percent transfer over to the baby. That's what I carry, and that's where it's kind of tough knowing that I'm not the cause of it but it was something I had that's basically the result of the loss. (Russ)

If an answer can be found regarding why this happened, then the chances of it happening again may be understood and treatments offered. Many losses are simply spontaneous and random. This information may help you make informed decisions, as this mother found:

> I was on bedrest by fifteen weeks with my first one for dilating early and preterm labor and you know, so I was just terrified that it was going to happen again. (Shannon)

If you have a medical condition such as diabetes or high blood pressure, then you may well stand a better chance of successful pregnancy if you take the advice of your doctor to stabilize your medical problem before you embark on another pregnancy.

The current recommendation is that all women of childbearing age should be on a supplement of 0.5 mg of folate before becoming pregnant. It is well known that taking the contraceptive pill can reduce your folate level, so waiting for a complete cycle after ceasing the pill may be helpful.

You may be contemplating another baby if your previous baby was born with special needs—for example, a congenital defect, chromosomal abnormality, or a metabolic disorder. An important step may be seeking as much information as you can before you make the decision to try again.

> One of the issues that we talked about was taking the risk to have another child. And several of the parents who had normal children first and then a child with disabilities commented on the joy and balance in their lives and how Tom and I did not have that balance. Our life was very intense; very intense. (Jan)

You may not ever find a definite answer as to why your baby died. This can be difficult and challenging. Even if you are given a cause, you still may not know why your baby died. For example, most babies who are growth restricted live. So you might ask, "Why did my baby with growth restriction die?"

ARE WE READY YET?

You may have had a plan in your mind for your family even before you ever became pregnant. For example, you may have wanted your children to be close in age so they could be playmates, or you may have wanted a set number of children before you turned a certain age. The death of your baby may have interrupted those plans. Now may be the time to revisit your plans, realizing that there may not be a schedule you have to adhere to.

> We didn't have the mindset that we have to get pregnant right away. We just realized the plan isn't ours. We're just going to live our lives and whatever happens, happens. That took us a long time to even think that way. We just felt so cheated by the loss. We felt like if we don't have any control, we will do what we want to do. (Clare)

If your last pregnancy was high risk, fraught with problems, and needed extensive hospitalization, you may have to anticipate the same with a new pregnancy. Thus, you will need to consider how this might impact you, your partner, your employment, and/or your other children.

You and your partner may feel like you are always having the "are we ready yet?" conversation. This can feel endless and exhausting, especially if one of you feels ready and the other does not. If this is the case, a helpful technique might be for you and your partner to agree on *when* to discuss planning your next pregnancy. Women and men may often have differing ideas about when to try again. For women, the biological need to have another baby might be overwhelming, whereas men have said that because they do not share the same physical connection as their partner during pregnancy, they feel their parenting begins only after the birth of their baby. So the loss of a parenting opportunity may feel more recent for them.

> It's when you're able or mentally ready to have a baby again. I guess we both knew each other very well or were in tune with each other. We really didn't discuss "Are you ready?" We just kind of knew that we were both ready to try again. (Allyn)

Some couples might struggle with sexual intimacy in the aftermath of their baby's death. This can interfere with achieving a new pregnancy. You may also find solace and reassurance in reconnecting sexually. Differences in desire are common, especially if one of you is more focused upon achieving another pregnancy. The key is for you and your partner to communicate with one another.

HOW LONG DO YOU WAIT?
Once you have made the decision to go ahead, the next decision you need to make is when. There is no right time to try again. The most recent research says that there is no difference in outcomes in delaying a pregnancy after loss.[2] However, each case is individual, so you should always discuss your specific situation with your health care provider. Sometimes a doctor will advise waiting if your loss came further along in your pregnancy, to give your body a chance to heal and prepare for a new pregnancy. If you were further along, it may be some months before you are even able to become pregnant again.

> We asked the doctor what the best time was medically for us to wait to make sure she's healed up. They said for her, she'd be fine in a month or two. But they

recommended that we wait at least one cycle for her to make sure everything's working again, and she was okay. (Allyn)

It is important to consider that having a new pregnancy during the same months of your previous one can also be difficult. If you become pregnant soon after your baby died (especially three months after), then your new baby will be born at the same time of year as the birth and death of their sibling. Think very carefully about how you might deal with such a situation: Will it be a celebration for you? Or will it be a difficult reminder? Just being aware of how you feel can help with your planning.

It is also important to give yourself a chance to physically recover from the pregnancy and have time to grieve. Regardless of the timing of your decision, and even if you think you are ready, you may be surprised to realize that missing and longing for your deceased baby will continue.

We decided that the time was right for us when we had more hope than fear. That happened to be six months, actually, and I got pregnant the first month we tried. So it was a nice surprise. (Kim)

Questions to ask yourself about your readiness to be pregnant again:

- Are there triggers for you that may set off an avalanche of emotions? For example, seeing another baby, or a pregnant woman, or walking past the baby food at the grocery store?
- Do you have the resources to cope with a pregnancy that might be physically and emotionally challenging?
  - Do you have the social support to do so?
- Is your body ready for a new pregnancy?
- Is your partner ready for a new pregnancy? What about your children?
- Are there any lingering doubts or medical concerns you need to address?
- Does the gender of your new baby matter to you? If yes, there are some resources available.[3]

FERTILITY, INFERTILITY, AND BODY CLOCK

You may have concerns about your fertility and be conscious of your biological clock ticking. Particularly if you are over the age of thirty-five, you may feel you do not have the luxury of being able to wait to feel more ready be-cause you might know that you are at an age when your fertility will decline and the risk of genetic disorders will increase.

You may have had difficulties getting pregnant previously, or perhaps your pregnancy was the result of infertility interventions. There are some things that may boost fertility naturally, such as reducing stress, staying a healthy weight, and increasing physical activity.[4] If you are having difficulty getting pregnant, particularly if you have not had trouble before, it may be appropriate to seek help from your maternity care provider.

If you have experienced infertility before, then achieving pregnancy again may not be as easy as just deciding to try. The expense, along with having had previous losses or a menstrual period you did not want to have, can drain you of energy or even sap your desire to try again.

> There is often so much disappointment in the infertility journey—procedures canceled because conditions turn out to be suboptimal, procedures that don't end in a successful implantation (someone in our group said, "I feel like every period I get is a devastating, red banner of failure"), procedures where im-plantation is initially successful but can't be sustained, and procedures where pregnancy results but is quickly lost. (Jerri)

OTHER PEOPLE

Other people might have been affected by your baby's death and might be giving you all sorts of unwelcome and unhelpful comments or advice. This can be hurtful and exhausting, no matter how well meaning. If you feel you are having difficulty facing other people, it may be useful to find someone you trust who will quietly listen and help you deal with unwanted comments.

> At times I've worried about getting criticized for getting pregnant so soon. You just kind of worry about what people think. The biggest thing that I've had to hold onto is: you have to do what's right for you. We knew what was right for us, and this is what it has been. That part is what I wouldn't want anybody to forget or lose sight of; that you do what's right for you and it's different for everybody. (Deanna)

SUMMARY

As you move forward in trying again, remember: love for your deceased baby remains in your heart. This will not change once you are pregnant with a new baby. It is important to keep talking to one another or to share your journey. These reflective questions may help you get started.

REFLECTIONS

- Do you think you are ready for another pregnancy?
  - What issues have you considered together (with your partner and/or loved ones) that have brought you to this decision?
- Have you discussed your pregnancy plans with your proposed maternity care provider?
- What would your deceased baby want you to know as you consider having his/her sibling?

As we relearn the world, we give lasting love for those who died a place within the larger context of our lives. No matter how important those who died and our love for them have been, we did not, nor do we, give our hearts to them alone. Not only must we struggle to let go of their physical presence and long-ing for their return, but we also need to let go of any singular, sometimes pre-occupying, focus on them and their absence. We need to let go of loving only them to the exclusion of any others. . . . We love those who died when we go on without them by our sides, with lasting love for them in our hearts and with our hearts open again to the wonders of life on earth.[5]

3

Beautiful Chaos:
A New Beginning

Conception to Twelve Weeks' Gestation

After achieving pregnancy, one mother described her feelings as "beautiful chaos." In your ongoing grief, you have risked trying again. Excited to be pregnant, you also know pregnancy carries no guarantees of bringing a living baby home. Instead, the promise of a new life is mixed with feelings of joy and fear. At the very least, you may have ambivalent feelings, if not unadulterated fear.

> It was all emotions all at once. It was instant joy, but it was also intense fear because it's like, okay, there are so many things that can happen. (Teresa)

> The day that I found out I was pregnant it was like a good pain. I can't say I've enjoyed the pregnancy, like last time, a beaming mother-to-be, so happy and naive and everything, and this time, even though I'm so ecstatic to be pregnant and carrying a baby, we hope that this baby lives. (Deanna)

Depending on how long you have waited or been trying to get pregnant, you might start to feel like you've been pregnant forever. You are likely to be feeling a full range of emotions. Happiness mixed with fear is normal. Your loss of naivete causes you to never take pregnancy for granted again. This can be very unsettling in your life and your relationships. You may be constantly checking, and with every ache and pain you may fear the worst.

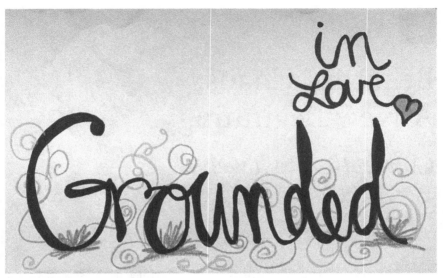

Courtesy of Diana Le-Cabrera

Totally unexpected, a new layer of grief can surface even if you feel well supported in your grief—for example, in an infant loss group or by a professional counselor—and thought you were ready.[1] Instead, this pregnancy is a reminder of your deceased baby, and you realize this baby could also die. This does not mean you did not do your "grief work" to prepare yourself to open your heart to a new baby. You are focused on your deceased baby more than wanting to acknowledge you have a new baby growing. It is important to remember that even parents who have healthy children first are always, understandably, more focused on the child they know, their living child. In your case, it is the deceased baby you know best.

> It was hard. I was very happy to be pregnant again and I was completely terrified. I was maxed out with stress about what would happen, if I could deal with it. And, of course, at the same time I was carrying my grief with me. It goes without saying that being pregnant again did not alleviate any grief at all. It just added a whole layer of complexity to that. So the first part of the pregnancy I was just keeping my figures crossed and trying to get day to day. (Kate)

Even if you are carrying this fear and anxiety, you may still be hopeful.

You always have the thought of a good outcome, you have hope, and you want to think positive. Let's be realistic here. Our only realistic time last pregnancy, the realism of it was he died. This pregnancy is kind of still a hope. (Len)

Following your initial reaction, a whole host of emotions can surface, from fear of another loss to guilt over what happened last time. You can worry that you are worrying too much and even feel angry at putting yourself through all this again. Many parents talk about feeling guilty: guilt that they did not recognize that something was wrong with their pregnancy, or even guilt that they did feel something was wrong but did not act in time or could not get their concerns heard.

I felt scared that I was going to go through the same thing. Constantly guessing what my body was going to do and if I was going to be able to hold on to the pregnancy, blaming myself, a lot, for what happened before. I just felt a lot of guilt. Then I just started getting mad at myself for even getting pregnant again. Why would I do this again to another baby when I couldn't hold on to her [previous baby]? I felt I could have changed my pregnancy with her because I knew in my gut the whole time, I knew something was wrong, but I kept ignoring some clear signals. I'd go into the doctor, but I felt like I didn't shout loud enough with her, so I felt this tremendous fear and guilt that I wouldn't be listened to. What if the same thing happens?—tons of feelings that were so scattered that I was not like myself at all. (Diane)

Anxiety will ebb and flow. You may think your anxiety will go away after a certain point in the pregnancy but be assured that living with anxiety is part and parcel of a subsequent pregnancy. If there is a pregnancy-after-loss support group in your area, it may be helpful to join it. There are also online groups that you can join.[2] Keep in mind, however, that hearing stories of other people's losses can also be upsetting because you will learn other ways babies can die.

FEAR OF MISCARRIAGE

In your previous pregnancy, if you even thought about the risk of miscarriage, you never thought it would happen to you. But now you realize miscarriage is more common than you'd thought. So you might now be feeling vulnerable and constantly checking for signs.

I was afraid every time I went to the bathroom. I called a friend of mine who also had losses: we call it the "fear of the wipe." That every time you go to the bathroom you're going to see blood. That was my whole pregnancy—every time I went to the bathroom, even after I got through to twelve weeks. (Marybeth)

At the moment you may not be feeling all that lucky. You are not denying that you are pregnant but may not be able to "go there." There is probably little that anyone can say to reassure you. It is a matter of weathering the storm. You may feel tentative and realize the hopes, dreams, and expectations of a long-term future with your new baby may not come to be. This is a protective measure to cope and does not mean you do not want and love your new growing baby. You will cautiously move forward, one day at a time.

Your entire pregnancy is tainted by the sadness you feel about your previous loss, on top of the anxiety and fear that you may lose another baby as you now know from experience that infant loss and stillbirth can and did happen to you. You can no longer enjoy a carefree and excited pregnancy like those who haven't had a tragic loss before. However, there's also a bit of joy in feeling that resemblance between the two pregnancies. (Ana)

You could indeed have some bleeding, so be mindful, but this may not necessarily mean the end. Check with your maternity care provider to find out what is going on. There are many causes of bleeding other than miscarriage, as these parents found:

There was one point where I was bleeding a lot with Jack, and I was convinced, "Well, here we go again." And it was a cervical polyp or something. So then for a few hours I thought, "I'm never going to have a baby." (Dawn)

All the stuff just trying to get pregnant in the first place and then having a pregnancy that seemed to be going okay, but she had a fair amount of bleeding, and right away you're thinking it's another miscarriage because we had experienced two before. It was just nonstop. Sometimes it would kind of clear up for a number of days and then it would come back. We went to the emergency room once. There was just always that issue. You're just always stressed, and every day that nothing happened, you're "whoopee." You still have that clenched stomach, but a little bit of a sigh of relief. You go through not knowing how things are going. But the baby still seemed to be doing alright. (Mark)

If you are worried about having another miscarriage, it might be useful to have a plan of action about how you might cope if this happens. The plan might involve a maternity care provider that you trust and not being in the same room where you previously received bad news.

> I bled at seven weeks. I called the doctor. I'd been with her for fifteen years, and if I was going to get another miscarriage diagnosis I wanted it to be her. But I wanted it in a different office than where I found out about the other miscarriage. I thought, "I can't go back in that room because if I go back in that room they're going to find the same thing." Then she said, "You guys—look, she's fine." To see this little seven-week baby and see the heartbeat that looked totally fine, and then to go back at nine weeks and see it again, I knew that everything was going to be okay and that she was fine. But I still worried. So, I attached right away, but it was just that worry was there. (Marybeth)

DECISIONS ABOUT A MATERNITY CARE PROVIDER

You will need to decide about who will care for you during this pregnancy. Will you decide to stay with the person who cared for you last time, or will you change? Many parents feel comforted and reassured being cared for by someone who knows their story and who knew their baby. However, others, who might have had a bad experience, may find rebuilding trust in their maternity care provider too difficult and will wish to change. This mother explains her reason for staying with the same maternity care provider:

> She was so great; she was so respectful of the losses. I think a lot of physicians might not even talk about that or acknowledge that, because you know how some people are: "Well, they were first trimester." But she was so great about it. She couldn't find the heartbeat right away. And I thought, "Well, I'm twelve weeks, and I haven't bled, and I know everything's fine." And then she looked on the ultrasound, and the baby was fine. I still had some worry until I could get to twenty [weeks] and get the level two ultrasound [morphology scan] and make sure everything was okay. (Maryjane)

Here are the thoughts of another mother who changed her maternity care provider:

> Because of my first son's death, I knew that I wanted the umbilical cord monitored. I picked this new OB because she listened to me. Other doctors were like,

"Well, basically it's rare, you'll be fine." The one I chose listened to me, and said I could come in anytime I wanted to come in and check the baby. She was accessible all the time, which I really needed. I still had to convince the MFM [maternal fetal medicine] to monitor the umbilical cord; they weren't so gung ho about it. I basically had to reassure them that I understood things could still happen. You can't see the whole cord at once, but I said, "If you're not looking, you're not going to see something, so you really have to look, and then we can decide what we are going to do from there," and they agreed. (Danielle)

You may have lost trust in yourself, so when considering who will care for you, find someone who will respectfully listen and act on your concerns. This is important, especially if you feel your concerns were not heard the last time or you feel you ought to have known something was wrong.

The reason I didn't trust myself was because with both losses I felt like I should have known what was going on. (Lydia)

The first visit to your MCP is likely to be an anxious one. It may be helpful to take someone along who will be supportive. Tell your maternity care provider about your fears and concerns. One perinatologist suggests telling your MCP up front that you are going to be scared and that they should not take it personally. Together you can create a plan for your pregnancy, including timely and appropriate referrals where necessary. Your care provider can give you reassurance, but always ask what objective data they have to confirm as much as possible that the baby is safe at this point in your pregnancy. You need objective data because you are so subjectively involved.

LOOKING OUT FOR YOURSELF

It is natural to feel helpless and vulnerable, but you can also be empowered to take control of what you can control. You may want to do everything you can to achieve what's best for you and your baby. Don't be afraid to ask questions of the health professionals caring for you.

I had suffered and wasn't able to bring any children into the world and felt that I'd earned the right to be direct, to be specific, and to let them know what I needed. (Marci)

Even though the doctors might say there's no reason to believe that anything's wrong if you had healthy children in previous pregnancies, you know there are no guarantees.

> After the second loss, I asked for the antiphospholipid antibody and they weren't going to do it.[3] I went to lunch one day with my good friend who is a perinatologist, and she brought me all these articles and said, "You need to give these to your doctor. I really think you should get these six tests done and give them to her." Almost two months later, I think, "Oh, she must have thought these articles were okay." I'm sure she read them because she always does what she says she's going to do. And I get to the office and here's this message: I think I want you to have these tests. And everything was negative, but at least then I knew that. So that helped me feel a little bit better, that maybe this can still happen. (Marybeth)

It is common to want to change things to be as different as possible from the last pregnancy. You might consider changing your lifestyle, work practices, diet, and level of exercise.

HIGH RISK

Your pregnancy may not be viewed as high risk by some care providers, even though you have suffered the death of a baby. However, in light of your loss, you deserve to know that concerns will be taken seriously. Inform your maternity care provider about what they need to do while you are still in these early weeks; for example, without needing a full appointment, you may just need to go in to hear the heartbeat for reassurance.

> The first trimester went really fast, actually. Everything was going really well. Being at MFM [high-risk] clinic where you get seen more, there's more testing, there are ultrasounds every time. Just from a medical standpoint this gave me more peace of mind, in terms of knowing that things were okay, knowing that they were going to look for different things because of my history. (Kim)

Even if you don't have any particular complications, it is helpful for your MCP to recognize that you will have certain periods, such as getting over the time when your previous baby died, when you will be especially anxious. It can be helpful to make plans for that day so you will not be caught off guard.

In order to cope with this difficult time, your doctor may suggest additional tests and screening.

CHECKLIST FOR YOUR PRENATAL VISITS

The MCP caring for you will need to know as much as possible about your previous loss and what you think you might need to help you through this new pregnancy. One doctor said, "If you weren't paranoid during your next pregnancy, I'd be really worried about you."

The following box shows a checklist that you might like to follow in outlining your plan of care for the pregnancy. Change or add to meet your needs.

Prenatal Visit Checklist

First Visit 8–12 weeks	• Discuss your emotional needs and how you can best be supported. Include your current level of anxiety, ambivalence, or excitement. • Tell your MCP whether you want them to mention your last baby. • Give the MCP times when you might be especially concerned, such as anniversaries, particularly if you are at all worried about how you are going to cope with them. • Consider whether diagnostic testing including CVS and blood tests are needed and when these will be done.
Subsequent Visits 12 weeks	Fetal Heart: Ask to hear it as soon as it can be heard if this is an issue for you.
16 weeks	Blood Tests: Ask your MCP for full information on the risks, false positives, and outcomes of each test prior to testing.
18–20 weeks	Ultrasound: Organize support for yourself; ask about the possibility of a video.
24 weeks	Discuss your baby's individual movement patterns.
28 weeks	Remember to go to sleep on your side from now on.
32 weeks	Ask about a birth plan form or write your own.
36 weeks	Discuss plan for birth with your MCP. Talk about a debriefing tour and how to address this step as well as suitable support people who might accompany you.
38 weeks	Ask about fetal monitoring for reassurance.

DIAGNOSTIC TESTING

First trimester diagnostic testing may be offered to you, such as chorionic villus sampling (CVS).[4] This is a test done under guided ultrasound where a tiny sample of placenta is removed by needle biopsy. The results give information about genetic abnormalities. Before undergoing the test, consider how you might respond to the results. For example, if they come back negative for an abnormality, that may be reassuring, but if positive, then you may face more tests and difficult choices. You may decide the potential risks are outweighed by the benefits. However, deciding to go ahead with diagnostic testing should be a decision you make with complete information between you, your partner, and your MCP after a full and frank discussion involving all risks and potential benefits.

> [My husband] sees a lot of kids with genetic disorders. He was pretty clear that he wanted me to have an amnio. I was unwilling to do it because the point of having an amnio early is so you can do something with the results. I knew that I wasn't going to terminate this pregnancy. I'd done that before, a couple times in my early twenties. I just wasn't going to do it unless we find out there's something fatal to the baby or to me. (Kellianne)

YOUR UNBORN BABY

You may have already heard about the impact of stress on the unborn baby and be worried that your stress is causing harm. However, research tells us that pregnancy is a natural state of raised cortisol levels (stress hormone).[5] We don't know whether stress in pregnancy has any negative effect. It is important to remember that your unborn baby is sharing the same space that your deceased baby did and is also feeling your emotions. The scant research done on children born after loss suggests these children learn about grief while carried in the uterus of grieving mothers, and many see this as a gift from their deceased sibling.[6]

> I was really worried that I would somehow infuse my anxiety into my daughter. That her life would be forever ruined by my anxiety; that somehow, she would be a nervous child, a nervous adult. None of that has come to pass, but it was very real at the time. (Lydia)

In the first trimester you can feel out of control, but one of the things you have control over is how and when you share the news. Bereaved parents often don't share the news of their new pregnancy.

Feelings of sadness are rarely understood by family and friends who are hoping you will "be done" with your grief. It can be hard to share the news with others. Be ready for other people's reactions. You do not want to hear "everything will be fine this time." Decide together as a couple who you will tell in case you do need support in the event of another loss.

> I think, especially for the first trimester, we kind of both held our breath, didn't share with very many people at all that we were expecting. People that we did share with, we just asked them to keep us in their prayers, stuff like that. (Diane)

> People need a lot of compassionate friends who are just going to listen and not tell them how to do their pregnancy or raise kids, because they don't know: friends who will be quiet and listen. (Lydia)

SUMMARY

Even as you may hold back embracing a new pregnancy, your unborn baby is growing and "becoming." By the end of the first three months, your baby will be at a very young developmental stage. Keep in mind that this is the same baby you will see at birth. All the structures and organs are present but need to develop and mature. Figuring out how to think about this little one as a forming person can be hard.

Sharing your thoughts can be scary. In the book *Tears Change Us*,[7] the author writes that times of chaos can be a way to reflect on your feelings: in this instance, your grief for one baby while anticipating the birth of a new younger sibling.

REFLECTIONS

- What sorts of things can you put into place to help you through these early weeks?
- Which MCP will you choose? What questions will you ask?
- Think about who you might want to know about your pregnancy for support in these early weeks.

Uncomfortable Truths: Conflicted Feelings

Twelve to Twenty-Four Weeks

Nature never repeats herself, and the possibilities of one human soul will never be found in another.

—*Elizabeth Cady Stanton (1815–1904)[1]*

You have made it through the first trimester! This can be reassuring in that you are still pregnant, yet thinking of the weeks ahead can be daunting. Your loss of innocence has changed your meaning of pregnancy. You may not have symptoms of feeling pregnant as you did in the first trimester (e.g., morning sickness, overly tired). You may still feel tentative about this pregnancy.

> It's weird. It's like there's this bubble that I've created around myself that some-times is stifling because it feels like I'm being really negative about the preg-nancy. At the same time, it's comforting that it's there, like a protection. (Stacy)

SHARING THE NEWS OF YOUR NEW PREGNANCY
When and how you share the news with others will likely be very different than your previous pregnancy. You are fine waiting, keeping the news to yourself and your partner until you are further along to protect your emo-tions. Others may think a new pregnancy means you will stop grieving, but you want to continue to remember your deceased baby.

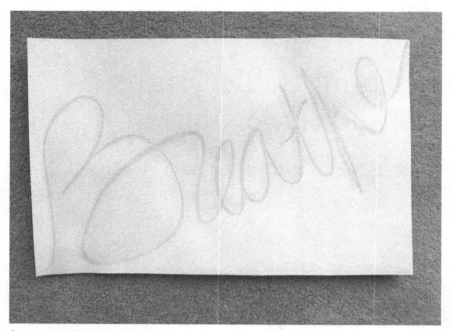

Courtesy of Diana Le-Cabrera

When I was pregnant the first time, people would say, "So, how are you doing?" Nobody did that the second time. They were pretty cautious, afraid I was going to cry or lose it or not want to talk about it, which was true. So we didn't talk about that we were pregnant. (Diane)

Making a full commitment to embracing your pregnancy can be hard. You don't want to hear unhelpful comments such as asking whether you want a boy or a girl. You probably just want a healthy baby. If you are in a second subsequent pregnancy after having a healthy child, you also don't want comments from others who have no clue about your history.

Is this your first? What are you having? Oh perfect. You'll have one of each. And I want to say, no, actually, I already have a boy. I always say, this is my third child. (Danielle)

Another big concern in telling others is not wanting to hear their excitement when you are still feeling so fearful of the outcome. You may decide to only share with friends who were supportive around your loss, as they probably have a better understanding of your mixed feelings.

> The anxiety, exhaustion, thinking of change, not wanting to talk about the pregnancy, it's all normal. I have one friend who literally did not want to acknowledge that she was pregnant to anyone. She barely told me, and then said she didn't want to talk about it. So we didn't! (Christine)

You may also feel hopeful. You want this baby and are trying to stay positive. You want something to feel normal, like anyone announcing their pregnancy, and enjoy the same feelings of support and happiness that you felt the first time around. Regardless of when and with whom you share the news, you have control and can choose when it seems appropriate. It might depend on when you see family members.

> We waited to tell my grandparents and the rest of our family. I think it was probably about fourteen weeks, mostly because I was going home for a weekend and would see them in person. But we were definitely going to wait until after that time to tell everyone else. (Kim)

Remember, no matter when you tell others, expressing your specific needs for emotional support will help others know what they can do to help during your new pregnancy. This gives you some sense of control when you are feeling so vulnerable. And it gives others specific ideas for things they can do to be there for you.

OTHER PREGNANT WOMEN

Even though you're now pregnant, it may be too painful to be around other pregnant women. Perhaps they are having a second or third child, and you feel left behind. Perhaps you're still worried about your own situation and also worry for them.

> You see women walking around the mall just "oh so happy I'm pregnant," and it's like "Do you know that you don't always end up with a seven-pound, healthy baby in your arms? It's just not that way." (Sheri)

We have many friends who are having first babies, second babies, and we saw them going through pregnancies, not a care in the world, no worries. And I couldn't believe it. They were incredibly naive. I felt angry about it, and jealous. (Katie)

Hearing others talk about their pregnancies or babies can also be hard. It's not that you are mean and uncaring. You want to be happy for others. If you can, let them know it can be hard hearing their stories, while still being happy for them. Be clear about what you may need from others around baby issues.

My best friend was expecting her second child. I told her that just because something bad happened for me doesn't mean I'm not happy for her. There have been times when it was hard to hear our HR director at work talk about her grandson, who would be the same age as Hope. I didn't want her to think that she couldn't share her joy. (Deanna)

AIMING FOR A HEALTHY PREGNANCY
You may still feel ambivalent about taking care of yourself. Your goal is to try to stay emotionally, physically, and spiritually healthy. Get enough rest and relaxation and try to eat a healthy diet. Discuss with your health care provider a safe level of physical activity to maintain. Do the best you can, knowing you can't control every outcome.

It wasn't until my body started changing that I completely let myself get a little bit excited about it. (Kim)

When you find tensions mounting, remind yourself to take the pregnancy day by day, hour by hour, or minute by minute as necessary. You may find it helpful to write an early pregnancy plan with your health care provider, knowing plans can change during the pregnancy. These do not need to be long and may be quite simply expressed, as these two samples demonstrate:

This is our second pregnancy. Our previous baby, "Daniel," died at twenty weeks' gestation for no known reason. Although we are thrilled to be pregnant again, we will need a lot of reassurance in this pregnancy that all is well. We would like to come in more frequently for heartbeat checks until we get past twenty weeks' gestation. We may still be scared and want to renegotiate our plan of care at that time. Please let us know what more we can be doing to make sure this baby is okay. We had no birth preparation before and so cannot bear going to a regular birth class. We will need a special birth class as we get closer to our due date.

This is our fourth pregnancy. Our third baby, Ashley, died four days before her due date. We thought everything was going fine until we went in for what we thought would be our last appointment and found out on ultrasound scanning that she had died. We will be nervous when we have ultrasounds in this pregnancy. We are very hopeful all will go well but are still frightened. We need a lot of reassurance throughout this pregnancy as to *why* you know the baby is safe. We will also need help talking with our other children, who are three and five. They do not understand why their sister died and have already asked if this baby will die too.

CLOTHING

Most women will start to wear maternity clothes from eighteen weeks onward: a way to proudly announce to the world that they are pregnant again. As your unborn baby grows, expanding your uterus, you can no longer deny or avoid thinking of a baby within despite your fear of another loss. Maternity clothes take on a different meaning, a constant reminder of your loss. The idea of wearing the same maternity clothes from last time can be very difficult, and you might choose to throw them away or borrow from a friend, as this mother did:

My best friend just had her second healthy baby. I'm going to ask her if she will let me use her clothes. (Joan)

Your partner can also find it hard to see you in the same clothes. This is something you might want to discuss together.

Every time I see her in that dress I am reminded of our dead son. (George)

I was really angry, so I threw out all of the maternity clothes I wore with Jude. I had a bathing suit that I wore when I was pregnant with Jude. I saved that because it was really nice and I remember being happy wearing it with him. It was just the one thing that didn't make me angry. I wore it, and my husband did not want me to wear it. He said, "Could you get something else?" I didn't think that he'd have the same feelings toward some of the clothes, but he did. I got all new clothes for Arrow [first baby born after Jude], which I'm wearing now [her third pregnancy], and a few new things now to fit me because I've been pregnant four years in a row and keep getting larger and larger. (Danielle)

Purchasing new clothes may also be something helpful that your friends and family can do for you. If you have older, healthy children, you may feel comfortable wearing clothes you wore during their pregnancies.

I feel okay using the same clothes because I wore them with my older, living sons. (Julianne)

HEARING THE HEARTBEAT

During these weeks you may need to visit your clinic often "just to hear the heartbeat." Discuss this as an option with your health care provider, taking your health insurance into consideration, where applicable.

I'd heard of some woman that had gone through a pregnancy after loss where her doctors had let her come in for a weekly heart monitor check. So I asked my doctor "Will I be able to do that?" He said, "Oh sure. Anything you'd like, we can do that. You don't need an appointment, we'll get you in." (Rochelle)

You might be tempted to buy a device to hear your baby's heartbeat (fetal stethoscope or Doppler). However, listening to your baby's heartbeat at home cannot be substituted for medical advice. The presence of your unborn baby's heartbeat is not a sign of fetal well-being. For concerns about your baby's well-being, you need to arrange a visit to your maternity care provider without delay.

GENETIC TESTING

You may not have had access to CVS earlier in your pregnancy, so you might be offered a diagnostic test called amniocentesis, a prenatal test in which a small amount of amniotic fluid is removed from the sac surrounding the baby.[2] This procedure can be done any time after the fifteenth week. This kind of testing can help you make a more informed decision about your baby's health care. Going ahead with this test should be a choice made between you, as parents, and your doctor, after you have all the information you need about risks and potential benefits to make an informed choice.

> We decided not to do any extra testing as whatever happens is meant to be. I prayed for a healthy child. (Kathy)

Even if your previous baby died because of a genetic condition, you may choose not to do more testing, and that is fine, too. You may decide that you will follow the course of the pregnancy through to its natural conclusion, whatever that may be. It's a personal choice.

> We didn't do an amniocentesis. We very intentionally said that unless something would indicate that for a medical reason—discernment—we needed to have one, we were fully committed to this pregnancy and would not do anything to my body or her that might potentially disrupt it or just even violate my body, like sticking a needle in my belly. (Cheryl)

Your partner may disagree with your choice of testing. It is important to share each viewpoint to make an informed decision.

> He was clear that he wanted me to have amniocentesis. I was unwilling to do it because the point of having an amino early is so you can do something with the results. I knew that I wasn't going to terminate this baby. I'd done that before a couple times in my early twenties. I just wasn't going to do it unless we find out there's something fatal to the baby or to me. So, having not done that early screening, I am eager to do the ultrasound and know that everything is okay. I believe that everything is okay. (Kellianne)

ULTRASOUNDS

The trauma of your previous loss will increase your anxiety during certain points in your pregnancy. An ultrasound examination is one of these points. Around eighteen to twenty weeks' gestation it is common to have a detailed ultrasound (level II, anomaly scan), which provides more comprehensive information on your baby's development at that point in time.[3] It is important that you are well prepared for this scan. Make sure your MCP has sent over your records and history so the MFM (maternal fetal medicine) clinic has a chance to review them and knows your story.

Entering the space of an ultrasound will bring back memories of your deceased baby. Both you and your partner are likely to be very emotional. This may be when you learned your baby had died or had an abnormality. Let the technician know your history before you enter the room. Ask to see the heartbeat first.

> The first time, I just thought to myself, "The last time I had one of these put to my belly I saw my child dead." And I just thought, "It's not going to be that way this time." There he was all moving around and perfect, so. (Sarah)

> For somebody who doesn't have any medical training: I'm lying there, I have no idea what I am looking at, the ultrasound technician maybe is aware, by the file, that I've had a loss, but that isn't really her priority to care about that. She would start checking for the regular things, like checking a foot or a head, but I'm lying there holding my breath, trying to read that screen to figure out if there's a heartbeat. So I learned to say, in a way that I felt comfortable with at the beginning of every ultrasound, "I've had a loss. Can you please tell me as soon as you can if the baby's alive?" which was hard to do without crying. (Katie)

Even after birthing successful, healthy babies, anxiety around ultrasounds is very common. Many couples find they have a conflicted relationship with ultrasounds.

> It was petrifying. Even with all of them [three healthy children after her first loss]. I'm absolutely terrified of ultrasounds. I feel like I'm going to throw up. It's awful. Some people just love ultrasounds, love to see the baby, see the baby moving; for me, ultrasounds are awful. (Dawn)

If you had a previous preterm birth, your doctor may do earlier ultrasounds to assess your cervix. A cerclage may be put in place if you have a diagnosis of cervical insufficiency (weakening of the cervix).[4] There may be other tests or monitoring suggested if you have other complications. Discuss these with your partner and maternity care provider.

> I was watched every two weeks with ultrasound, and at twelve weeks they noticed that my cervix was shortening. Then at fifteen weeks I had a cerclage because it was shortening even more, and I was having the same symptoms I

had with Anna, just sooner. I wasn't having the bleeding, though, but the other physical [symptoms]—the back throbbing, the tightening—I started noticing earlier. Then I had the cerclage, and about probably eighteen weeks I started going in because the tightening was a lot more frequent. (Dina)

Ultrasound technology offers helpful information for parents to make decisions. Keep in mind, however, that there are still many limitations to the knowing and understanding that it can offer to you. It is important to work with a team of professionals who are experienced and trustworthy and who listen when you voice concerns.

ULTRASOUNDS AND GENDER

The ultrasound technician may be able to identify the gender of your baby. Let them know whether you want to know your baby's gender.

We don't want to know the gender, so they avoided that area. We want it to be a surprise. Only Derik knows [deceased son]. That's really a neat thing to say because I do envision Derik a whole part of this thing, too. (Susan)

We didn't want to know the sex of this child, but that request did not get to the ultrasound technologist. We now know we are going to have a son. I wish I did not know that. (Kathy)

You may wish for the same gender as your deceased baby, or you may not. Both feelings are perfectly normal. Even those who have not experienced a loss sometimes have a preference; for instance, you may feel you can only be parents to a certain gender.

I found out it was a girl, and I walked out of the clinic on cloud nine. It helped me relate to the person I was growing inside me more as a person. And I think it did help me bond with her because now I had the future images in my head of what she might like to do, or her personality. (Kim)

LOYALTY ISSUES

Around eighteen to twenty weeks, having more awareness of this baby as separate from your deceased baby, loyalty issues can surface. You are beginning to feel flutters and can no longer deny there is a baby growing inside.

You may struggle with conflicting feelings. You want to love and embrace this unborn baby, but you also want your deceased baby back. When you first feel your unborn baby's movement, learn the gender, or see an ultrasound picture, you can feel very strongly that you are expecting the "wrong" baby. These feelings are normal. You may also be grieving, for a time, the loss of the girl or boy you wanted.

> When I was pregnant I struggled with the feeling that we were replacing Lily. Having another girl such a short time after made it feel like it was just one really long pregnancy. I had thoughts often of "Now I'm really going to get my daughter," after which I would immediately hate myself. (Lauren)

> I couldn't tell anybody; I couldn't talk to anybody. I felt horrible—really guilty. I finally got this blessing of a child. How can I really care what sex it is? That seems so shallow. Yet I just couldn't get past it. I just finally had to accept the fact that this is just what I'm feeling and that's just the way it is. I can't feel guilty on top of feeling bad about losing my girl. But now it's starting to sink in that I'm thrilled. I guess I'm starting to just go totally the other way. (Shannon)

It is important to remember that your loyalty right now is to the baby you know best—your deceased baby, the baby you still long for. As movements become stronger, you will begin to learn who this new baby is as a separate person.

ADVOCATING FOR YOURSELF
The loss of your previous baby has changed not only the meaning of pregnancy but also you as a parent. This has made you more aware of advocating and sometimes even fighting for what you need.

> After having three losses I earned the right to be direct, to be specific, and to ask for what I need. (Marci)

Even if you have had a successful pregnancy since your loss, you may still want to be considered high risk and followed more closely.

> With this pregnancy, I feel like "oh, you have a living child." We don't need to be so worried and uptight about this pregnancy. So they are a little more relaxed in the care this time. But I'm also forty. (Danielle)

Advocating for what you need is important. It is your body and your baby you are working to keep safe.

> One other thing that was helpful for me was learning how to advocate for myself in a different way, because I had such different needs, to try and temper my stress, my anxiety. I cried through every appointment with the subsequent pregnancy. But once I was able to start doing that, it was a good step for me. I really had to let doctors and nurses know what I needed for my anxiety and worries. (Katie)

JOINING A SUPPORT GROUP

Joining an infant loss support group with other bereaved parents may have been part of your journey through loss. A pregnancy-after-loss group can be an important resource for you now. There are both online and in-person pregnancy-after-loss support groups. Other parents can reassure you that all your feelings are normal.[5]

> We continued to go to the infant loss group for the first weeks of our pregnancy. It wasn't really real for a long time, so we fit better into that group. I wasn't really there yet. Then at eleven weeks I thought, "We belong in the other group now." (Clare)

In this pregnancy, the journey is about your new unborn baby, a sibling to your deceased baby.

> Once we did go to the group, we realized we needed to change gears. That made it more real. Okay, we're pregnant again. Last time we got to sixteen weeks and we're not there yet. It felt like forever to get to that point. (Mike)

> I liked that the group focused on the new baby while also letting us grieve for our deceased children. (Beth)

> My pregnancy-after-loss group served as my anchor during Eliza's pregnancy. My due date seemed so far away, I could not count the weeks or months. I could, however, count down the seven days between group meetings—that was a manageable task—and I looked forward to spending this time with women who would allow me to voice my scariest thoughts in a safe, supportive space.

Sharing my fears helped to take away their power. I left each group feeling loved, encouraged, affirmed, and hopeful! (Katie)

In a pregnancy-after-loss group, you join other bereaved parents who share the story of previous babies and similar feelings you may have of fear to attach to your unborn baby.

I needed to meet and talk with other women who understood what I was going through. I felt like I was completely alone. No one in my family had ever experienced the death of a baby at term. Even though they tried to be supportive, I felt isolated and like I was going crazy. Support groups helped validate my feelings and experiences. I knew that others had gone through similar losses and that they were feeling lots of the same things. If they could survive it, so could I. (Lauren)

Sharing your interwoven feelings out loud, grief for one baby and attachment to your new unborn baby, can help give a place to both of these feelings. Sometimes you can't say things because you don't want to start crying, so the words actually can't come out because your crying stops them. It's really important to get past that and verbalize what's going on so your thoughts don't get hidden.

I didn't go to the pregnancy-after-loss group until I was about five months and I started to have contractions and I got really scared. Then I started going and it was incredibly helpful. It was wonderful support, really helped me get through those last four months. I think saying things out loud is huge. There's so much about honoring that and what's happening and what you're going through. (Mona)

I became a regular online support group member when I was put on bedrest for our PAL [pregnancy after loss]. It was hard not being able to physically go to a support group, so having the online option was a godsend. To me it felt like a sacred place and time that I could set aside just to talk about our son, Owen, and my grief, as well as my worries about the pregnancy with others who could empathize. It's important to have an outlet for all those emotions or you truly feel like you can't cope and may burst or fall apart when your grief is triggered.

In the beginning I preferred one-on-one therapy; then I got into attending support groups. (Ana)

LGBTQ+ PARENTS

If you are in a same-sex relationship, you may find your experience of loss is a common denominator in a support group discussing issues of your next pregnancy. You will find caring support that can benefit you.

> One thing that was different was to ask for help. On top of worrying about my feelings after our daughter died, I worried about whether I would be accepted because I am lesbian. My partner and I decided we just had to be "out" so we could get the support we needed through such a high anxiety time. After the first couple of support group meetings, I felt fine. Everyone was very open, and we all shared a common thread of having our babies die. It was no different for us as lesbians; we still had the same feelings that other members had. I felt so supported through the next pregnancy; I don't know how I would have made it through without the help of group members, professional staff, and the wonderful caring and sharing we did. I still keep in touch with members of the group for support in raising our new daughter. (Grace)

Of course, like a loss group, you learn all the many ways babies can die. But you also learn what others are doing with their care providers to keep their babies safe. This can give you more information to learn how to advocate for you and your baby.

> I think what I got most out of the group was speaking with the other mothers. They would talk about their care and what they asked for and what issues they had. This educated me on what I should be asking and looking for to keep my baby safe. One woman had lost her child with the way the cord was inserted into the placenta, and she went on to explain what she needed to look for and what I needed to ask for. (Danielle)

A well-facilitated group helps support your continued bond and parenting relationship to your deceased baby while learning ways to engage with your new unborn baby. Most comforting for you may be sharing your deceased baby as an important member of your family with other parents as they support you in this new pregnancy.

REBUILDING TRUST IN YOUR BODY

Your level of trust never gets back to where you were. Even with healthy older siblings, you may have lost trust in your body as a safe place to grow a healthy baby. However, this doesn't mean that you can't work to rebuild trust.

> One other thing that grew and grew as the pregnancy went along was that my body didn't feel like a safe place for this baby. I remember looking back thinking about my first pregnancy with Max—the healthy happy pregnancy—I didn't have a worry in the world that it wouldn't turn out okay, even Alma's (deceased baby). I felt that when I was carrying Max I was keeping him so safe and warm and lovely in my stomach. Now, with this pregnancy, I felt like my body could turn at any moment and I had no control over any of it. It was really scary and awful. I couldn't understand how I went through a pregnancy not terrified. (Katie)

Rebuilding trust takes time and effort. You already know you can't control the outcome. What you can control is how you care for yourself and the baby. Try to remember each day what you are doing to nurture and grow this baby. Keep a journal of the ways in which you are nurturing yourself and your baby. Forgive yourself immediately for small transgressions. Don't be too hard on yourself for days when you are not perfect, no one is.

> Neither one of us want to talk to this baby. It's hard. Last time I talked a lot more to Nicolas. I'd sing to Nicolas in the car. But at the same time, we don't want to rob this baby of anything we did for Nicolas. Steve had wanted to read to the baby all along. I said, "When we see this baby, then I'll know more that things are okay, and then we'll start." So at nineteen weeks we started playing baby Beethoven every night, and we read the baby a book every night at bedtime. (Debbie)

ANXIETY

Your anxiety can ebb and flow depending on what is going on. There are many proven methods for dealing with anxiety. Perhaps yours is mild and some meditation and quiet thoughtfulness is enough. Perhaps you need to speak with a therapist or other trusted professional. Being part of a faith community is also helpful. Give yourself permission to feel anxiety and to manage it as best you can.

> You're paranoid, I think, no matter what in any pregnancy, but I think when you've lost one you have a lot more paranoia. Yet you try not to be negative and have a lot of anxiety. At least for myself I worry when I read different books. Some books say any anxiety is normal, but if I have too much anxiety, I'm wondering if it's going to affect the health of my baby. Always in the back of my mind: "Is this baby okay?" (Katie)

When fetal movements begin but are not yet regular, you may experience an increase in your anxiety. Never hesitate to go in to your health care provider when you are anxious for reassurance that your baby is still alive. And utilize coping skills to help you minimize how often that might be.

> This time I pay more attention to what he's doing and what my body's doing and how I'm feeling, and if anything's just weird, I'll call and ask to be seen. I don't get stressed out about it too much, but there's always almost like an itch inside, a little stress that wasn't there before, since I found out I was pregnant. (Sarah)

Even with objective data that all is well, you can continue to feel anxious until your next appointment.

> Every Wednesday I go to the doctor and I'm thrilled. Everything's fine. By Thursday, I'm not feeling so positive any longer. By Friday, I'm really not feeling it. By the following Tuesday, I'm a basket case. I don't sleep. I'm anxious. I'm cranky in the morning. I can't even get to it fast enough because I'm convinced every single time that by Wednesday, when I go in there that morning, the baby is going to be gone. Now it's gotten a little bit better because I can feel the movement, so I'm not as anxious because I've felt the baby move that same morning. (Debbie)

COPING WITH ANXIETY

If you have a family or personal history of an anxiety disorder, you might want to seek more support. Doing so may help you understand whether your anxiety is just fear of another loss or something in your history that is more complicated and may need to be treated. It is important to know whether you have any type of trauma that could be triggering strong emotions that are interfering with your daily life. If this happens, you may want to consider finding help with a therapist who has experience in processing trauma during pregnancy.

> How much of this anxiety in this pregnancy has everything to do with Finn and our grief and how much to do with our family history? (Katie)

> I was pregnant and having anxiety attacks. I just relived that whole hospital scene. I'd be driving and I'd have to stop the car because I'd start crying, or lose it. I needed counseling during that time. (Diane)

> We found a wonderful therapist who guided us through our grief and our next pregnancy. (Christine)

It's also important to remember that some things are just not within your control. Mindfulness meditation may be one practice to help you with those feelings of not knowing what might come next. There are some useful and easy smartphone applications (apps) you can download to help you with managing your emotions during this time. Other resources, such as massage, acupuncture, yoga, or other types of complementary therapy, can also help you cope with your fears and anxieties. Find what works best for you. Encourage your partner to also reach out for an activity that can help with stress, too.

> I was introduced to yoga through another loss mom, a few weeks after we lost our daughter Sonum. This loss mom told me that "trauma release" and "restorative" yoga helped her with her loss. Yoga and meditation have allowed me to feel how close my daughter is to me and feel that eternal bond a child has with its mother. I now have the yoga instructor come to my home every week in my new pregnancy with my unborn baby boy. (Shaylee)

> I had therapy and acupuncture throughout, to try to keep me calm. I was at the high-risk center weekly. Having twins just added another whole layer of anxiety, trying to monitor both of them throughout. (Debbie)

If you conceived using reproductive medicine and had failures, you may still be struggling with believing a baby is growing inside. It can be helpful to find a resource to lessen your anxiety that also supports your wish to fully embrace your unborn baby.

When I found the CD, I not only used it faithfully, alternating it with a Healthy Pregnancy CD from Health Journeys and listening EVERY night at bedtime, but I shared it with every woman in my infertility group who got pregnant after me.[6] The women who used it felt that it accomplished three important functions: (1) on the initial listening, it relaxed them and provided a calm, quiet time when they could reduce their stress in support of their pregnancy—something we had been well-trained to look for from our mind-body class; (2) it provided a constant reminder (using the language of "baby" versus "fetus" or "embryo" or something euphemistic or medical) that we were, indeed, pregnant and had taken the step from needles, test tubes, specimens, and clinic procedures, to a living baby; and (3) it helped us realize and accept that our baby (babies for our multiples moms!) was no longer a dream—no longer some distant, seemingly unattainable goal. It was the real flesh and blood infant for whom we had so desperately wished, prayed, hoped, and worked, and they eagerly needed for us to shower them with all the love we dreamed of showering on them, for us to talk to them like we dreamed we would talk to them, and for us to bond with them the way we dreamed of bonding with them. (Jerri)

Sometimes, because of your history, just acknowledging anxiety and grief as a given will help.

I talked to one PAL mom recently, and she said that it actually helps her if she just embraces and recognizes her grief. Then she finds that her anxiety decreases compared to when she is trying to push the grief away. It made a lot of sense to me, though I'm sure everyone is different. (Christine)

If you can, try sharing your feelings out loud with your baby, giving reassurance that your anxiety is about keeping him safe, not that you are afraid to love. When you feel ready, try beginning a journal, or simply write a poem, as this mother wrote in her early weeks of a new pregnancy:

A New Life

A new life has formed in me in this place you used to be.

I am happy and excited but with some difficulty.

My feelings conflict so often and are mostly bittersweet.

I'm not sure if I'm strong enough should history repeat.

I know the joy of giving birth, and I know the pain of death.

I feel so out of control sometimes, it's hard to catch my breath.

I wonder if this baby knows how torn I am inside,

struggling with my grief and feelings that I hide.

I want this baby to know it's loved without reservation.

But I keep my guard and defenses up for self-preservation.

I love this new little one as much as I love you.

I know I have room in my heart for this baby too.

It's just that it's so hard to let myself get too attached

when I can't control any outcome; the future or the past.

(Used with permission from Ann Dean, mother of Bailey)

GETTING TO KNOW YOUR UNBORN BABY

As you come to the end of your second trimester your unborn baby is also exploring the intrauterine environment, flexing and extending body parts, practicing movements. During these weeks your baby is also hearing voices, thus learning about the world he is being born into. This makes your baby more real, and you may begin to pay more attention, even this early. As you live with the fear that this baby may never be born alive, you may also realize pregnancy may be the only time you might have with your baby and that you are already a parent to this baby.

> I just take more time out to focus on the baby and the pregnancy; now he's really starting to move a lot, so that's helped a lot. Sometimes I just pray: "Give me a sign that it's going to be okay." (Jan)

In spite of not knowing how her pregnancy might end, it is important for this mother to enjoy every moment with her new unborn son:

> This time I know that I just cherish every day I have with him, that he's moving and he's kicking. I think I'm even more excited to meet him. I want to know if he looks like what Owen looked like. I just want to take care of him better and want him to be okay, to see him, and bring him home. (Sara)

SUMMARY

As this unborn baby begins to make his or her presence felt within you, this may produce feelings of disloyalty to your deceased baby. If you can, try writing to your deceased baby about the sibling who is coming. This may help you understand that you are a parent to two babies.

REFLECTIONS

- What would your deceased baby want you to share with this new unborn sibling?
- What do you want to tell this new baby about his or her deceased sibling?
- Remember, you do not have to give up loving one baby to open your heart to another baby.

5

Viability: Balancing Hope and Fear

Twenty-Four to Thirty-Two Weeks

This chapter will give you information on coping skills that other parents have found helpful. You will also read more about prenatal testing of the unborn baby's development that can be offered any time after twenty-eight weeks, depending on the reason for your previous loss.

During these weeks you begin to balance the hope of bringing a baby home with the fear that something may still go wrong. If your previous loss was before the unborn baby was "viable," you were aware during the loss that your child would not survive. Now, at this stage, if you should happen to go into premature labor, your baby has a decent chance of survival in a special-care baby unit or NICU. So, as you move into these weeks, you may feel and act less stressed, and your family and friends may misinterpret this situation and think you are now okay and "coping," when actually what is really happening is a new and different phase.

> In two weeks I will be twenty-six weeks along, and I know at that point if there is a problem we can deliver her and she will have a good chance of survival. So to me, getting to that point, I take it day by day. Any day, week, month that she's still here with us, it's just a miracle. (Rochelle)

FIELDING QUESTIONS

At this stage you cannot usually hide the reality of your pregnancy from family, friends, and even strangers in the street and shopping mall, as your belly

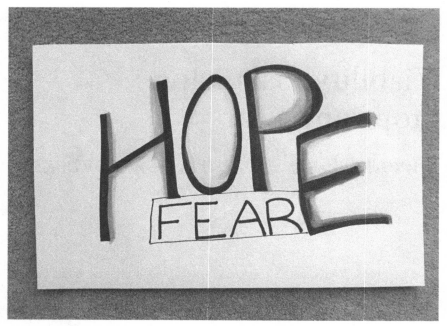

Courtesy of Diana Le-Cabrera

is likely beginning to grow and become round. This may mean that you face unwelcome and difficult questions such as "Is this your first baby?" Preparing ahead of time for those common questions can help.

> When people would say things like "when the baby is here . . ." I would respond, "Yes, fingers crossed." When I did talk about my pregnancy, I would say, "If the baby is here," or "Assuming that all goes okay." (Christine)

THE DREADED QUESTION

You could probably count the number of times in this pregnancy that people asked you the question you dread hearing: "How many children do you have?" Even if you have rehearsed your answer, it can still catch you off guard. Some moms want to include their deceased child in their responses. Others don't wish to make the questioners feel uncomfortable. Knowing how you want to answer can make it easier for everyone.

Your partner may also struggle. Often, the partner feels he or she needs to protect the pregnant partner and let people know they have more children to honor their own feelings.

I guess everybody goes through real tricky situations when you see people, and they see you're pregnant. They're real happy for you, and strangers ask you if it's your first kid, and just getting a good answer for that without it being a downer is hard. We went out for dinner and saw somebody I knew from work, and his wife was pregnant, too. She said, "Oh, is this your first?" And then, here it comes: "Oh, no, not really. We had two girls last year and they lived for two weeks. So this will be our third." You see the looks on their faces and don't know what to say because you kind of caught them off guard. When people ask Stacy, she'll say it's complicated and won't go into it with them. But I like to tell them what happened. (John)

These sorts of questions are often asked without thought, as a way of starting a conversation. The person asking doesn't realize that this apparently simple question might be difficult for you to answer. After all, you should know whether this is your first baby! It can be helpful to have a discussion on how to answer this kind of question with other bereaved parents. What might be natural for one person to say may feel unnatural or awkward for another. You may simply want to say "no, this is not my first baby," and change the subject. You may also stop and say to yourself, "Do these people really want or even deserve to hear my baby's story?" or wonder whether this person can handle hearing your story. You may decide what to say depending on the person who is asking. Certainly the person at the checkout doesn't need to know. Other times you don't share and may feel guilty not including all your children. You might solve this problem by saying something like "I have one living child with me and one who is in heaven."

MOVEMENTS

During these weeks your baby's movement patterns will gradually get stronger and more regular. This can be reassuring but also stressful. No longer in your mind are you just "pregnant." Your baby lets you know his presence by his movements.

Particularly when I first started feeling the babies, I was describing every single time I felt it and what it was like, and is that okay, until I got used to it. It's really hard to describe what you're feeling. I've sat there with information on preterm labor numerous times of the day and read through the list. (Janelle: twin pregnancy)

Once you begin to feel consistent movement, you may worry if your baby has a quiet period. You may wonder, "Is this enough movement?" Keep in mind all babies have sleep-wake cycles, so it is normal for them to have intermittent periods of being asleep and being awake. Usually these run in twenty-minute cycles, but some sleep cycles can last as long as forty minutes.

It's just the last few weeks: getting past the point of if I went into labor early that they might not be able to save the baby. I'm more able to understand when the baby's moving, and then I can start feeling where its head is and where its different body parts are. I'm starting to let myself get excited about being pregnant. It's not just a mechanism for me to know that the baby is alive and okay. I'm starting to have fun with it and appreciate it. (Maria)

Every time the baby moves it makes me smile inside, and every time the baby doesn't move, of course, I'm scared. And that's the point now. That's the roller coaster I'm on now; constantly worrying and wondering about the baby. (Deanna)

Most babies will settle into a fairly predictable pattern of movement by about twenty-eight weeks, such that you will know when to expect them to move and what triggers that movement: this may be certain sounds or certain activity that you are doing. For example, you may realize your baby moves a lot when you play certain music or when you are lying down to go to sleep at night. Getting to know your little one and what is normal for them is more important than getting a set number of movements in a given time period. Learning your baby's pattern is important, so give yourself time and space to connect and learn your baby's patterns; this allows you to note any changes to immediately report to your health care provider.

Definitely always in the morning—I just lay there in bed for fifteen to twenty minutes; it's just our time together. His relaxing time then may be between four and seven o'clock, until about a half hour after we've eaten supper. And then he's pretty active the rest of the night, until I go to bed. He's really starting to move, so that's helped. (Sarah)

If my husband begins talking to her—"Can I have a kick?"—sometimes that may take a while, but for the most part, he usually gets them, so that's good. I feel blessed to feel that movement. There are some times when I've been in bed, actually, and trying to sleep, when I'll switch sides or something like that: "Please settle down. Let's go to bed." Then I'll catch myself: "But I'm really glad you're moving." Because that must mean it's her way of telling me she's okay. (Kim)

You can try keeping a log of movements so you don't miss changes in your baby's usual routine, especially if you are busy with an older child and feel like you didn't pay close enough attention with your previous baby.

One of my fears was of missing any movements from the baby. I was haunted by the memory of my son, Anders, and his last day alive. I had felt him once in the morning, but looking back I think he was already under duress. I wasn't going to let that happen again. I started keeping a log of movement. It was life-saving for my anxiety. Every time the baby moved, I would check my log. A lot of times I had a note that the baby had just moved an hour ago or less. (Kari)

If you learned after death that your previous baby died from a genetic anomaly, this can be one explanation as to why your deceased baby's movements were not as strong as your current baby's movements. This may help you compare patterns of movement, sometimes giving you some reassurance that this baby is healthy. However, always remember that every baby and pregnancy is different, so you shouldn't compare between the two. If your pregnancy this time around is a lot like your previous one that ended in a loss, you might feel like you are also assuming the worst this time around.

Owen never moved a lot. I could never feel him move when I was standing up or walking, and I hardly ever felt him move when I was lying down. If I was on the couch and sitting still, he would move and be active and I could feel him. But this little guy just moves all the time and I can feel him walking, doing the dishes; throughout the day I feel him. And I never felt that with Owen. I just think Owen's little body was working so hard to keep that blood going through that he didn't have the energy to move as much. And he didn't have enough fluid to really move much at all. So, it's different. (Sarah)

This baby kicks a little bit more, so, okay, maybe this baby's going to be a fighter, a little bit stronger. Hey, everything's going to be okay. But I know that can all change fast too. (Rochelle)

You may have been told by your MCP that you have an anterior placenta.[1] That is when the baby's placenta is attached to the front wall of your uterus. Your MCP may also tell you this is a reason why you may not be feeling movements as soon as someone whose placenta is attached at the back. While an anterior placenta can make it a bit harder to feel your baby's initial movements because your baby's body is cushioned by the placenta lying at the front of your stomach, it's very important to understand that once you know your individual baby's pattern of movement, any concerning changes should not be attributed to you having an anterior placenta, as this is not a plausible reason for you to suddenly not be able to feel movements that you could before.[2]

STRESS AND ANXIETY

Of course, it is perfectly normal if you feel more anxious in this pregnancy, and you may need more attention from the professionals working with you. Never feel like you are being a burden to your care provider. They are there to support you and your baby for a healthy outcome.

I had a dream that the baby died. It was two days later, and I just couldn't shake it. Then one morning, I was getting ready for work, and I started crying in the shower and I couldn't stop crying. I called my mom and talked with her for about half an hour and then calmed down. I was just self-talking myself through it. They told me at the beginning, if I ever needed to come in and have a quick ultrasound and know that everything is okay, I could do that. So that's the one time when I called and went in without an appointment. I had Dan meet me there. So they hooked me up, and she happened to be sleeping at the time. "Why isn't there any movement? Oh, there's the heart, it's pumping away." I needed to see that she was still alive. (Kim)

Learning ways to cope with your stress and anxiety is important. What works for you may be very different from someone else. You may need to work with a therapist or social worker. Meditation and light exercise might do the trick for you. Seeking out other mothers in similar situations may also help alleviate some of your anxiety.

> If the baby doesn't wake up right away that's when I start panicking that something's happened overnight that I didn't know about. I can get myself pretty worked up by the time it does start moving. If it's early morning, I'll just sort of roll around. I'll get up, go to the bathroom, kind of shake things up a bit. I find that if I sit up in a reclined position, then it will start shifting around and start wiggling around a little bit. (Maria)

IF YOU ARE CONCERNED

Along with getting to know your baby and immediately going in if you have concerns, you need to pay attention to symptoms that might indicate all is not well with you or your baby. These signs may include pelvic pressure, excessive itchiness, increased vaginal discharge, bleeding, contractions, and decreased fetal movement. If you have any of these symptoms, you need to go to your MCP more frequently for reassurance that all is well.

> I couldn't feel Leah moving. I called and said, "I'm scared. I think she has died." And the nurse said, "You need to come in and get objective data because you're so subjectively involved." She sat me right down, monitored me right away. I could see the heartbeat; I was reassured, and we could go home. It's okay; she really is okay. (Jan)

> When I first started feeling him move, just like the first little flutters, for a couple days I didn't feel him at all. The nurses said, "Come in, and you can take a look at him on the ultrasound." He was fine. He was moving all around; I just couldn't feel him that much at that point. It's just not worth it to sit here and be worried about this. (Sarah)

By twenty-four to thirty-four weeks, a time most vulnerable to preterm labor, you are already parenting your baby prenatally. You will want to report unexpected changes to your MCP, especially in fetal movement and uterine contractions. You need a MCP who can provide concrete information about your developing baby and who will understand and validate your feelings. Once again, remember that it is crucial for you to know what is normal for your baby (not necessarily "how long it takes for ten movements") so any change in behavior will be noticed and reported.

I tell it to every pregnant woman, loss or no loss, when the doctor tells you everything is fine, that's great, but why is it fine? Explain to me, what are you looking at? Why is it good? What does it look like if it's not good? I never thought of that, and it stuck with me. Obviously, with my friends now that know about my loss, they're worried about their pregnancies. So it's weird; I'm also trying to reassure them: "As long as you pay attention to your baby. Ask for what you want." Because that was me with Jude [deceased baby]: "Everything's fine. Great." And I'd leave not even knowing why everything's fine. I didn't know about cord insertion and all that stuff. (Danielle)

PRENATAL MONITORING OF YOUR BABY

Electronic monitoring (nonstress test[3] and the biophysical profile[4]) of your baby is done to validate the baby's development and well-being. For most parents this begins at twenty-eight to thirty-two weeks' gestation. The nonstress test measures your baby's fetal heart rate at rest and during times the baby moves: as much as possible, try to see the same person each time, because as they get to know you and your baby, they will be much more able to meet your needs.

By the time I was thirty-some weeks, I went in twice a week: once for the ultrasound and once to my OB's office for a NST. I tried to space them so that one was at the beginning of the week and the other was at the end of the week. (Christine)

When attending for tests, tell your care provider that you need to see, or hear, the heartbeat first. This will be the case for all pregnancies, not just the first one that immediately follows your loss.

We were understandably extremely anxious during our second subsequent pregnancy. Our doctor wonderfully made time for us and answered all our questions whenever he was available, and the clinic nurse also provided much support over the phone, email, and in person. Our experience with ultrasound techs, however, varied. Some were wonderful and sensitive and walked us through each ultrasound explaining what they were doing, what they were looking for, and if everything looked okay. Others had not read our chart beforehand and asked us if this was our first pregnancy. This is an extremely painful question to answer: "No—this is not our first pregnancy, our first baby was stillborn." (Christine)

You may feel that your body let you down the last time, so even with objective data, you will still be anxious and worried. This is normal. It is common for your partner to be nervous, too, but many men say they withhold their concerns because they do not want their pregnant partners to worry.

When we go to the doctor for ultrasound he's [partner] nervous but he doesn't act like it because he knows I am so much. He tries to be the strong one. But he tells me he really is nervous. "I think I'm really just as nervous. I just don't want to show you that I'm as nervous." He's a better optimist, I would say, than I am. He would say, "It's going to be fine. It's going to be okay." I know he still gets nervous. I'm the more cautious one, and he doesn't like to think that way. He just likes to think, "Yea, it could, but let's not think that it's going to. Let's just think that everything's going to be fine. You might as well not worry about it until we have to." (Diane)

ADVOCATING FOR YOURSELF AND YOUR BABY

Loss of control is a feature of pregnancy loss. In this pregnancy, aim to control what you can control by taking an active role in your health care. This includes working with your MCP to help you make the best choices to keep you and your baby safe.

Another thing that you can control is the position you go to sleep in. Current research supports going to sleep on your side from twenty-eight weeks onward. This is recommended because when you lie on your back, the weight of the baby and womb can press on a large vein that supplies the placenta and thus reduce blood flow to the baby. Research has shown that settling to sleep on your side from twenty-eight weeks reduces the risk of stillbirth. It doesn't matter which side, but go to sleep on your side for all episodes of sleep, including settling to sleep at night, returning to sleep after nighttime waking, and during daytime naps.[5] When following this advice, it is important to realize that everyone changes their position during sleep. If you happen to wake up on your back, don't worry; research has shown that it is the going to sleep position that is most important. Ongoing research is also being done on the relationship between the quality of sleep in pregnancy, including sleep apnea (pausing in breathing while asleep), and fetal outcomes.[6]

> They're supposed to move so many times in an hour. I spent a lot of time count-ing movements, lying on my left side. I had my own blood pressure machine at home. I took it three times a day, morning, noon, and then at night. It was a lot of stress to keep on top of it if something went wrong. I went to the hospital three times, too, thinking something was wrong. (Diane)

During these weeks, as your baby grows stronger, you will be paying atten-tion to your baby's movements and asking more questions at appointments. You need as much information as possible that all is being done to keep your unborn baby safe.

> Toward the end, about two or three weeks before we learned that she had died, I could see that the movements had started decreasing and the intensity wasn't as much. Could it happen this time around? Well, it could, but this time we're seeing the doctor more so they can catch anything. We're constantly asking questions: Is the amniotic fluid volume okay? That's one thing that had gone down significantly a week and a half before she died. The doctors are going to be watching this one carefully. I know we are in good hands and doing every-thing that we can. (Rochelle)

Even if your MCP knows your history, it can be hard to respond when someone does not understand what you need. It is important to have a MCP you know so that you do not have to repeat your history to new people. However, the provision of incorrect advice can fracture that relationship and can be challenging and exhausting. Unfortunately, not everyone is as aware as they should be of the latest research on fetal movement as an indicator of fetal well-being.

> I went in for one of my regularly scheduled weekly BPPs [biophysical profile] at thirty-five weeks. I was with a tech I hadn't previously met and had to repeat my history. When the tech asked me, "How has baby been doing? Have you been feeling him move?" I answered that while yes, I had been feeling movement, it

seemed to be less. The tech's response was utterly inappropriate and WRONG! She informed me that it is normal to experience a decrease in movement late in pregnancy. To which I responded that it is not normal and that she should not be providing outdated and incorrect information to pregnant women but should be encouraging them instead to seek care if they do perceive a decrease in movement. To that she appeared offended—for contradicting her professional opinion—and responded, "Well, that's what the doctors tell us to say." I told her that doctors can be wrong and not keep up with the latest information, especially when it comes to stillbirth. The latest research shows there should not be a decrease in movement and change should be reported. "It's normal" is what I was told the day before I found out my first son had died—when I called to report a decrease in movement. Then she said, "Ok, well, let's just change the subject." And after that last comment I was so shocked, hurt, and livid that I just became speechless! (Ana)

At twenty-six-and-a-half weeks, I didn't feel him. I woke up at 12:30 a.m. I had felt him around 8 p.m., before I went to sleep, and hadn't felt him since. I told my husband, I'm going to the hospital. I'm bawling, crying, I can't feel my baby. I explained my previous loss. The nurses were great. The doctor comes over and he starts lecturing me: "We don't really count kicks until twenty-eight weeks." I'm staring at him thinking, "Are you kidding me? As if I'm going to stay at home because it's not twenty-eight weeks." And then he tells me, "Oh, you don't feel the baby all the time." And I just look at him, and I say, "Yes, I know. This is my third child; they do not move constantly." He had no bedside manner. (Danielle)

Even when you do the right thing, you may have to stay strong to advocate for your baby. Nobody is more invested in your baby than you. Depending on how your previous baby died, you may ask for testing to begin before thirty-two weeks' gestation. For example, Ana's baby was stillborn at thirty-two weeks' gestation, and she was never given a concrete explanation. She did not want to wait until thirty-two weeks, so she asked her doctor to begin testing at twenty-eight weeks. Testing gave her a "baseline" of her unborn baby's development at that point in time.

MINDFETALNESS

Mindfetalness is a term used to help mothers be "mindful" of their babies.[7] This can be one way to help you cope with your anxiety as well as get to know your baby. Put yourself in a space where there are no distractions so you can focus on the intensity of your baby's movements: the way in which the baby moves and how much the baby moves. Questions to ask yourself are: Can the movements be felt distinctly? Are the movements of the same intensity as usual? Is the baby moving as much as usual? It is important to quickly report any concerning changes in intensity, pattern, or frequency to your MCP.

> I use meditation, centering, and stillness to assess my whole thought and what's happening. I'm trying to get a sense of separation from the babies, in the sense of their movements, where my body is and where their bodies are—just trying to locate where everybody is. And also think about a sense of connection with them. (Janelle)

Try communicating to your unborn baby. Your baby is rocking with each breath you take, hearing your heartbeat, feeling your worries and concerns, but knowing the worry is because of the baby who was here before, who you loved and wanted but whose life was far too short. Your stress and anxiety is not because you don't want this baby but because you want him so much.

> We talk to Ethan about Andrew. I talk to him the same I would have talked to Andrew had Andrew been alive. He needs to understand this anxiety is coming from other things, not him. (Audra)

You may be like this mother who throughout her pregnancy journaled to her son Jude, who was stillborn. In her second pregnancy, fearing getting too close to her unborn baby, she waited longer to start writing to baby Arrow (girl). Now in her third pregnancy, she is having more difficulty writing because she knows this baby is another boy. In her mind, she knows she can keep girl babies alive but is unsure about boys.

> I wrote to Jude until he was born. I put pictures of his sonogram in "You're So Big": Can you believe how much I love you and I haven't even seen you yet? So I continued to do that. I didn't give up on him. I still wrote to him—the things I did before he passed. When I found out I was pregnant with Arrow, I didn't start writing right away. I wrote maybe a little bit later. I didn't want to jinx it. But then I thought, "Well, if something happens, I wouldn't want this baby to think I didn't care about it as much as I did Jude." So I wrote to her as well. It's

weird, with this baby, Stone, a boy, I've only written a few times. I feel more superstitious but I can't get my head around, well, maybe he will live. So I have written to him, but it hasn't been as much. (Danielle)

GETTING THINGS FOR THE BABY

If your last baby died before you prepared a nursery, you may begin making steps to prepare. You want to have hope that this baby may be born alive.

I didn't furnish the room, but I bought things each month, and it turned out—not consciously on purpose—that was my optimism and hope. (Kim)

Alternatively, you may remember that you had nothing ready for your previous baby, so you may make a conscious effort to prepare this time as a way of parenting your baby.

We weren't going to find out the sex so I hadn't gone out and bought a lot of stuff. I kind of regret that. As a mother, I should have done that. Why didn't I go out and buy a little pink teddy bear? Things I had to do a day or two before her funeral because I wanted to put things in the casket with her. So now I'm going out and buying more. I just feel like this way I'm doing more to bond with this child. To me that's important. I'm going to do as much as I can, because what if she does pass? You hate to think of the terrible what-ifs, but you'd have to face them, knowing it can happen to you. (Rochelle)

You may want to wait until the very end of your pregnancy to make preparations, and that is normal too. You may also have had well-meaning people, thinking they were doing the right thing for you, remove everything you had ready for your baby who died. So in this pregnancy, you may delay all preparations for that reason.

The first pregnancy we got the room ready, doing all that. This time we did nothing. While I was in the hospital, they took down the crib, they took everything in the bedroom apart and bagged it up and put it in the closet. So when I came home from the hospital there was nothing there. They thought that would help me. I couldn't go in there, hold the baby stuff and cry. I told them that was a serious miscalculation, that they shouldn't have done that. I remember a week after I was home, after having the baby, wanting to go and cry in the baby room that we had set up that had been dismantled without asking me. So the next pregnancy I couldn't get ready because I didn't want them to do that again to me! I won't get ready this time. And I have nothing ready. (Diane)

CELEBRATING YOUR NEW BABY (BABY SHOWERS/GENDER REVEALS)

Parents who do not have your life experience usually start thinking about preparing for events like baby showers and gender reveal parties, now the norm in many places. You may not feel ready to make nursery preparations, which is often noticed by family and friends who may comment on your lack of preparation. Be reassured that, given your history, this is normal behavior. Family and friends may want to give you a baby shower, but this can be hard, especially if you had one for your deceased baby. You have control over whether you want a shower.

I do have my sister giving a shower with family and friends after my due date. I had a couple of showers scheduled, some that were going to take place prior, and some that were going to take place after Luke's birth. So this time I think we'll just do them after instead. (Kim)

You might consider solving this predicament by requesting family and friends to bring gifts unwrapped. The gifts are set out on a table for everyone to see and become a gathering of hope rather than just a baby shower.

I wasn't necessarily forced to have a shower, but three people had asked me about it. It is just too painful to sit there and open up gifts when you have no guarantee your baby will come home. We had some people that understood not to wrap anything, but some people did. I don't know if they didn't get the memo or didn't understand. I thought maybe I should [have a shower]. I need to do something about getting excited about this pregnancy. Go and rip the Band-Aid off one day and have some sort of excitement. It was very bittersweet. It was a rough day, but we made it through. (Brittany)

Another mother agreed to something only if her friends would bring offerings that included both of her children during the shower.

Tino died at twenty-two weeks, so we did not have a shower. My friends really wanted to do something, so I agreed and had a shower for Lucian that was ostensibly for him, but I invited only a small handful of people who I felt I had already shared grief with and told them that it was really a shower for Tino and Lucian because Tino never got one. I guess I treasure any opportunity where I honor Tino with others. The shower was a way to honor Tino and welcome Lucian and involve a small handful of friends in that process of welcoming one and grieving another, as the two are intertwined in my life. I asked the people at the shower to write a note to both boys, to Tino, who had died, and to Lucian, who wasn't born yet. It was very special to have five people that I am close with write to Tino in particular, to honor him in that way. Material object, a note; I will keep those always. Rereading those would be something I could do to give some time to Tino. (Karen)

SUMMARY

As your baby grows and movements become stronger, you may be more able to concentrate on this unborn baby who needs your attention now. Journaling during these weeks about the missing sibling can help you focus on your growing relationship to this unborn baby. As you work on learning about "fetal mindfulness," your baby is aware of when you touch and massage your belly; consider playing music that helps you relax with your baby.

Parenting:
One Baby Deceased;
One Growing Inside

Around this time in the pregnancy, many parents will have mixed feelings around who this baby will be as you continue your role as a parent to your deceased baby. Over these months you have been working hard, learning ways to advocate for your "inside baby" who needs your attention now.[1] You know that this new baby is not a replacement, but in your heart it can be difficult. This chapter has been written to provide you with helpful guidelines in seeing your babies as separate individuals and honoring your role as a parent to all your children.

> I can remember talking in group about separating these babies who were two different people. Even though they were in the same space they were not the same baby. (Joanne)

A DIFFERENT PREGNANCY/A DIFFERENT BABY

It is perfectly natural to wonder whether you can love your unborn child as much as you know and love your deceased baby. This is not unlike parents who have never suffered a loss and are having a second baby. They also wonder whether they can ever love someone as much as the child they already know. For you, your deceased baby is the one you know best. Your growing little one can feel like a stranger. Learning to love this baby will come as you begin to realize that continued grief for your deceased baby can walk alongside your attachment to his new sibling.

Separating this baby from your deceased baby can be a challenge. You may want everything to be different. Intellectually you know this "inside baby" is not your baby who died. Even when you know the gender before birth, confusion over separating your babies can continue.

> I was reading Carol Cirulli's book, in terms of bonding with this baby. Oh, gosh. You know, I didn't think about it in terms of parents who wanted it to be their previous child, who didn't even want to recognize this baby as a separate individual. I've never had those feelings.[2] (Kim)

> As soon as Emma died I really wanted to have another baby. I would always say it was not a do-over pregnancy, but I think in my heart in the beginning it really was something I wanted to do over, and I wanted it to be right because I wanted a little girl. We got pregnant and we found out it was a boy. When they said boy, I was so devastated. I didn't want a boy. I knew that wasn't appropriate and I felt really bad about it But I definitely came around; I became okay with it. I was actually happy it was a boy for the fact that I wasn't going to see a little girl grow up and spend every life episode thinking that it could have been Emma. (Sarah)

> I knew, intellectually, that he was a different baby when he was inside me but couldn't really tell the difference. I know there is a fear of attaching too much to a subsequent pregnancy, in case there is another loss, and I know some moms don't talk much about the pregnancy while other moms go all in and throw a baby shower, etc. I probably fell somewhere in the middle. If I could go back, I would probably try and pay more attention to the other differences between my pregnancies—what I craved, what I didn't crave, how I felt. But I do also think Jackson and Madison [deceased baby] were not that different in my belly. Once Jackson was born, it was easier to separate him from Madison because he was a boy. (Christine)

Risking attaching again takes time. A psychologist from Italy, herself a subsequent child, once shared the importance of parents understanding their subsequent children are conceived in grief. This may make sense to you. For example, the night after the memorial service was conducted, five months after the death of their deceased baby, one couple conceived their subsequent child. Their baby was conceived in a grieving womb alongside their love for each other. Don't be afraid to share your grief with this inside baby. This may bring you comfort, knowing your unborn baby is sharing the same space as their deceased sibling. There are people who believe your unborn baby already knows his missing sibling at some spiritual level.[3]

> Knowing my sons shared the same first home (in my womb) and behaved similarly was special since, even though they won't get to grow up together, I got to experience their similar personalities in utero, and I imagine they would have been very much alike if they were both still here. Of course, that then triggers the grief of not getting to see Owen grow up. However, there's also a bit of joy in feeling that resemblance between the two pregnancies. (Ana)

> The continued bond wasn't hard. I just sort of felt like his energy or his spirit, wherever he was, was bringing his sister along. (Danielle)

> I've thought a lot about one of the coolest things about subsequent children: you just think they were in the same space, and I always wonder if they knew that somebody else was living in there. I think they do. That's why it's important for me to let them know that Matthew was there, that he's their brother, and to celebrate his birthday, that it is a significant day and we recognize it. (Kate)

Even though you may realize your babies are sharing the same space, it can still be hard risking to attach when you can't believe this new unborn baby will be born alive. Different from your previous pregnancy, when you were feeling so emotionally invested, you may be trying to detach, fearful something dreadful may still happen. Until you hold this living baby, you may feel cautiously optimistic in order to protect yourself.

> I do think there's been a hesitancy to become as emotionally attached as I want to be because the pain of loss is deeper in me than I really realized. (Sarah)

> I definitely saw myself putting up walls in terms of cautiousness, not wanting to get too excited because people assume that everything is going to be okay. Once you have a statistic, you never assume that any thing is supposed to go the way it's supposed to go again. So I think I'd get excited but then kind of calm down and go, okay, well, just take it a day at a time, a week at a time, see how it goes. (Kim)

I definitely struggled during the pregnancies, but I also made a conscious effort to, at least some of the time, embrace them in case that was all I was going to get. E and C [names of the subsequent children] always knew about Sebastian, that he was the firstborn, etc. They would most certainly have felt sadness and anxiety both during the pregnancies and after their births. (Caroline)

As you begin to learn about your unborn baby's development at each stage of this pregnancy, you may be struggling to attach out of loyalty. Try to remember back to your deceased baby's development during the weeks of his pregnancy. Like your unborn baby now, you and your partner shared daily life with your deceased baby, however brief. If your previous loss was any time after twelve to fourteen weeks, your baby's structure was already formed, only at a younger developmental stage than you would see at birth. You may even have been able to hold this baby. During those weeks, your deceased baby had also developed skills: hearing your voice, your heartbeat, your love, already a part of your family environment. These memories honor and validate the life of your deceased baby and may help you understand that, however short the life you shared together, your deceased baby knew you as his parents. This realization may help reframe grief as your parenting relationship continues when others may be saying you hardly knew your baby. Today you are parenting two babies: one who has died and the unborn baby. Try to go ahead and risk embracing this new baby. Perhaps imagine this baby completing what your other baby began. You might imagine your deceased child breathing new life through this sibling. Whatever works best for you is okay. Below are some suggestions from other parents.

I think part of it was in reading about development and understanding that babies can start to determine sounds and listen and have the ability to hear at approximately seventeen weeks, I believe it is. That just kind of coincided with knowing her sex and that she could hear. It just made me want to start talking to her and sharing things with her, letting her know how much we cared about her. I can almost identify her with a name, and that sensitivity, I think, helped me with that bonding process. I read about a mom who said, "However many days this child has, whether in utero or out in the world, I want it to be of a high quality." That made a lot of sense. So whether you lost them shortly after birth again or whether you lost them whenever, you wanted to make sure that child knew who you were and that you loved them and cared about them and wanted to take the best care of them. (Kim)

GENDER: SEPARATING EACH BABY

In a previous chapter we highlighted how you may have felt when you learned the gender of your baby during an early ultrasound. As the time of birth grows closer, some parents will want to know the gender of the baby ahead of time. They feel this will give them time to process some of the emotional challenges they will face at birth. This is a different baby, a sibling.

> Russ didn't want to really know what we were having. But I said I have to know. If it's a boy I want to know because I have to prepare myself for that, the feelings that would come along with having another son and not wanting to feel like we're replacing the one we lost. (Rochelle)

> So mentally I had prepared myself when I first found out it was a boy. I didn't want to replace her, but I did have to mourn, knowing that I wasn't going to have those experiences with a little girl, that my time with her was short; I did have a daughter, but I'm not going to have a daughter that I'll put in first grade or go to her wedding. That was tough but wanting him to be healthy has kind of made that whole thing a little bit easier to deal with. The bottom line is: I really don't want to have to go through what I went through, losing a child for a boy or a girl. So it's been a little bit easier in my mind to put that to rest. I do mourn her, and I mourn what I won't get to do with her, but I'm definitely okay with a big healthy baby boy. (Dina)

You may still be struggling with gender issues, wanting the same gender again or wanting a different gender to differentiate completely. Or you may want something in this pregnancy to be a surprise and wait to learn the gender. Either way, you will have many mixed emotions at the time of birth, but mostly you will likely feel joy, relief, and happiness. As a couple, decide what will work best for you.

> So many complicated feelings, especially about the sex of the baby. Many couples will find out the sex if they did not last time and vice versa. We actually waited to find out for all of our pregnancies. My extremely impatient husband, who can't wait to find out anything, for some reason, wanted to wait to find out about the baby's sex. So, we waited. I think you are surprised whenever you find out. The downside of finding out at the end was that I had to process it while also processing the birth. (Christine)

What if we had found out in the delivery room? It's like you wouldn't have thought it was your kid. And I said, "No way. I'd have stood up on that table and said, 'That is not my baby. Someone across the hall with a girl has my baby—this is not right.'" It almost forced us to accept the fact that this is not the same pregnancy. This is a new baby, and regardless of all the precautions and all the paranoia, it is still a fresh start. (Shannon)

Conflicting feelings can also surface if you are having the same gender as your deceased baby. You may feel like one mother who did not worry when she was pregnant with her first subsequent child, a healthy daughter born after Mitchell's death. But this changed in her next pregnancy when she learned she was carrying another boy. She knew she could keep girl babies alive but was not sure about a boy.

I got scared when his due date was Mitchell's birthday. I started to flip out after that. I couldn't keep it together very well. I kept telling myself this was so ridiculous, but I couldn't make myself stay calm. I just worried about him. I had done so well with Johanna [first subsequent child], but knowing he was a boy just made me goofy. Then I started worrying he would be born on the same day, and I didn't want them to have the same birthday. Dave kept saying it doesn't matter if he's born on the same day, it'd be kind of neat. (Kathy)

REMEMBER: YOUR BABY IS ALREADY HERE

Despite worrying you will not bring a living baby home, as much as possible, try to consciously remind yourself that the "baby is already here." You have an awareness of this from feeling your unborn baby's movements: pay attention when your baby is more active and to when during the day the baby is active. Your "inside baby" has been learning about the world outside your uterus. He may already know the voices of older siblings, experiencing all the interactions you have with them, every book you read to them, and the places you take them. He may also know the voices of grandparents, if they are around, and people in your workplace.

I talked to him a lot about just how I was so glad that God was letting me have another baby. He moved even more than his sister, and his personality still shows that; the two of their personalities are so opposite. I read a lot to Johanna [big sister] and he was always there, too. (Kathy)

Pay attention to where the different parts of the baby are lying: the back (smooth), the limbs (lumpy), the feet. Feel the baby's body with your hands on your abdomen and the positions of the body parts changing. When do his body parts change as he moves about? Encourage your partner and older siblings to also get involved in learning your baby's positions. Notice changes over time of fetal movement or uterine contractions and the difference between kicks and the baby's total body stretches. It can also be helpful to visualize your baby rocking up and down with each breath you take—curled in a ball, moving gently, the same position your baby will need for comforting after birth.

> I was happy and excited that she was moving so much because she was so active. It was fun to see when her foot would stick out or something. I was off work for the summer, so I could sleep when I wanted to sleep. She was with me for exercise class and just was there. (Kathy)

> Now I know it's a daughter, unless they made a mistake. There's a bit of a face there to this little person. You can practically see the baby's fist poking out. We didn't even get close to that with Logan. We're looking forward to a normal, long pregnancy where we can experience all those things. (Mark)

> When he's excited, when he likes the music we put on or he likes the sensation of the bath, or when I'm just moving around. Hearing Patrick [older sibling] as well, he'll actually respond to that by being more forceful, and he'll also respond a lot to Morris's [dad] voice. Sometimes when I'm giving Patrick a hug, he'll wake up and move about. (Julie)

Your baby's movements may also remind you of your previous baby's movements. Remember, a pregnancy is a pregnancy, but one baby is different from another, and that can be hard for you to separate at first. And while pregnancies can be similar in many ways, having one end in loss does not mean every other one will end in loss, no matter how similar it might seem along the way.

> Feeling Jackson's strong movements often reminded me of Owen. It was hard to distinguish the two pregnancies, in that both babies were very active, constantly kicking and moving around. I would often feel confused wondering why

this baby would, hopefully, get to live and why Owen didn't get that chance if he had the same behavior in the womb. It triggered my grief remembering how healthy Owen was up to the night we lost him, especially because we were never given a reason as to why that changed, and he passed away so suddenly. As a parent pregnant after loss, my fervent hope was always that this baby would survive and we'd be able to bring him home, but that never replaced the feelings of anguish and remorse that we didn't get to do the same with his brother. (Ana)

Your wish to be happy can be overshadowed with grief for your deceased baby. You can feel sad that you didn't pay as much attention to your deceased baby's behavior in his pregnancy. Or that you didn't mark every milestone. That's okay. You had no idea how it was going to turn out.

We just feel like we owe it to this baby to be as excited as we possibly can. In a way, I feel like I'm trying to make up for the fact that I didn't put more emphasis on our last child. So there are feelings of guilt to try and make up for it. (Dean)

COMMUNICATING WITH YOUR UNBORN BABY

You may find it hard to share your feelings with this new baby. You have probably read or heard that the mother's stress and anxiety can have a negative impact on the unborn baby and worry about this too. While your unborn baby senses your emotions, it is important to know that this research has not been done with mothers pregnant after loss. It is okay to tell the baby your anxiety is not because you don't want this baby but because you want him/her so much.

I was really worried that my anxiety would affect my baby, that she would be a nervous person. None of that has happened. (Lydia)

It may be hard for you to share feelings with your baby because you are not as excited as you were in your previous pregnancy. Sometimes it can be helpful to put your feelings into words. Sharing thoughts out loud with your unborn baby can release pent-up feelings. This can be another step to help you know the baby as a separate individual.

I realized I talked to the plants as I watered them, so I decided I could do the same with my unborn baby, sharing my feelings. (Diana)

I just remember always just telling the baby, "You're your own person." (Sheri)

Knowing your babies are sharing the same space, you can also share the story of your deceased baby with your unborn baby.

I started having some guilt feelings about feeling really happy about this new baby coming into our lives. We had lost Sarah and yet we were happy for this baby. I apologized to him more than ever that I couldn't be happy right away. I told him about his sister. (Liz)

I think about Mitchell a lot, and I know she [subsequent baby] is listening. I was just so happy. I just could feel it was different. I felt so good. Her movements made me feel so calm. I loved it when I got woken up by her moving around. Mitchell's movement was like a fish in a fish bowl; I would only feel him a little. (Kathy)

As much as possible, try to enjoy each day with your baby. It is helpful to remember that if you try to hold back your feelings and this baby dies, you will grieve just as deeply as you did before. So you might as well go ahead and embrace this pregnancy and this baby.

Every time I get scared and fearful and want to disconnect, I try to think: "This is the only time he's going to be in my stomach; this is the only time that I have to connect with him this way, and I do not want to *not* be a part of that. I don't want to have regrets about this pregnancy because I'm still scared and fearful." I didn't buy anything for the baby until about twenty-eight weeks. Even that was a blanket. I finally bought clothes at thirty-two weeks. I didn't do any of those types of things, but I did try to mediate with him, connect with him. When I get scared, instead of closing him out, I try to connect with him now. No matter what happens, I want him to get as much love as he can from me, no matter what. I try to just say, "He's my son no matter what, and I'm going to enjoy this and spend time with him." I have all these other things in my head giving me the fear, and I try to tell myself it's going to be okay. (Dina)

I definitely struggled, but I also made a conscious effort to, at least some of the time, embrace them (twins) in case that was all I was going to get. (George)

Below is a guided imagery that can be a useful tool when you are trying to relax. Find someone who can read the script to you while you sit or lie comfortably, connecting with your unborn baby.

Settle back into your pillow/chair. Rest your head and body and sink into relaxation. Take a deep breath, breathing in . . . and out. Breathe slowly and purposefully, as naturally as you can. Let your emotions slowly release, bit by bit.

This baby you carry today has listened to your stories, has felt your pain, and knows your love is given cautiously, not because you do not love him but because you love him so much. This baby feels deeply the concern and protection you have clung to during this pregnancy to want him to feel safe.

Breathe in and out . . . visualizing this baby inside loving you and all the other voices in the family that your baby hears. This baby is waiting to come into the world to show you his own unique personality and will help you believe again that life can be good and beautiful. Continue to breathe in and out at your comfortable rate, letting go of as much of the fear as you can for this baby.

You have nurtured and cared for yourself and this baby all these long months. Now begin to allow your body to prepare for labor and birth . . . let go of the tension . . . let go of the fear. Let the contractions come when the baby is ready . . . start slowly and build up your strength, opening your cervix, allowing this baby to come out into your life. Let the children who came before celebrate with you this new baby who will begin to heal your wounds and nurture your continued journey into parenting.

REFLECTIONS/JOURNALING

Your deceased baby has already made you a parent. Think about the positive lessons learned from your continued relationship with your deceased baby. For instance, you may love more deeply because you have experienced the fragility of life. You have had to join the "club" of bereaved parents who understand the difficulty of your pregnancy and are your friends on this journey. List some of the new people in your lives who have helped you, both at the time of loss and in this new pregnancy.

SUMMARY

You don't have to give up loving your deceased baby to attach and embrace this new baby. Your bond and attachment is and will be lifelong. "Learning to love those who have died in separation gives them a new and welcome presence in our lives. We give their legacies places in our memories, practical lives, souls, and spirits. As we do, we realize how much of value in their lives has not been lost."[4]

REFLECTIONS FROM YOUR BABY

What Would Your Deceased Baby Want for You and His Unborn Sibling?

- He would encourage you to seek support from family, friends, support groups, and professionals when needed.
- He would want you to remember and cherish his legacies.
- He would want you to know he still loves you.
- He would want you to find your way back in life, embracing this new sibling while keeping love for him alive in your hearts.

Preparing to Meet the "Born Alive Baby"

Thirty-Two Weeks' Gestation to Birth

During these last weeks you may feel time is standing still. This has felt like a long pregnancy, but celebrate that you, your partner, and your soon-to-be-born baby have done it together. Of course, you feel scared, but you may have moments of hope and you relish your connection to your unborn baby. Over these many weeks you have learned your baby's movement patterns: when he responds to voices and maybe times he moves during the night when you wake up to go to the bathroom. Often you will see that these times may be the same hours your baby will wake up for feedings, already preparing you for life after birth!

MOVING TOWARD BIRTH

Staying pregnant can become very difficult. You want to "get the baby out while he/she is still alive." Will everything be okay this time, or will it happen again? You might even be saying to yourself, "I just wish I could go into hibernation and wake up having had the baby"—just like brown bears do! Coping with the last weeks and learning ways to deal with your anxieties can help you prepare for birth. Ask for what you need.

> I just needed to make it to thirty-seven weeks. We had permission to induce then and having a concrete end date gave me solace as my pregnancy progressed. As the weeks rolled on, my anxiety started to heighten, I decided I would do anything to get myself through. My doctor told me she would check

me into the hospital whenever I felt ready and they would monitor me until we induced. Having that in my back pocket kept me going. I had a seven-year-old and didn't feel like I could leave him for weeks as I lay in the hospital waiting. (Kari)

My doctors were open to induction after thirty-seven weeks, though we ended up scheduling closer to thirty-nine weeks. Both my sons came on their own (one at 37.6, the other at 38.3). This lack of control even in pregnancy is one of the hardest parts of parenting. (Christine)

You are in this together. Your partner can also feel it is hard to wait. During these last weeks, if possible, you might find it helpful for you and your partner to attend the appointments together. Then you hear the information and make decisions together. This can help in lessening your anxiety and give you both more information on when is the optional time to birth your baby.

I think this pregnancy will have seemed longer than the other because of the uncertainty of everything. Then from thirty-eight weeks on . . . because of the fact that the placenta often starts to degenerate, we think that thirty-eight weeks is term. Let's have it now. (Dave)

Try to think of other ways people around you might help you cope in these last weeks. For example, one father sent out a request to their friends, asking them to send signs of hope to help them cope with their increased fears and anxieties in the last weeks of pregnancy. They were overwhelmed with the wonderful responses and placed them on a wall in their family room.

Even if you have birthed a healthy baby since your loss and are in a second or third subsequent pregnancy, you can still feel anxious. In loving and watching your healthy, living child grow, you have a deeper awareness of what you lost with your deceased baby. Try to focus on the knowledge that you have been successful once, while continuing to seek reassurance that all is well.

My brain keeps saying I'm going to lose him because he's a boy [second subsequent baby]. I feel like I'm as focused as I was with Arrow [first subsequent child]. I think since I passed Jude at the finish line, as I advance in weeks my anxiety just gets more and more. Some people have a lot of anxiety from the

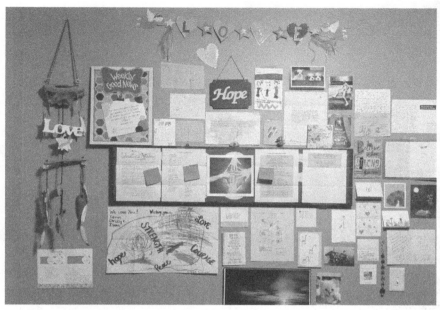

Courtesy of Kari Padin

beginning, and I think the more we get into the end of pregnancy the more chances there are he might pass. (Danielle)

Be open with your care providers about coping with your anxiety. During these last weeks you may need more appointments with your MCP. You are working hard to keep your baby safe.

Somehow the last few weeks seem to drag on even longer than the previous weeks. When I went into the hospital toward the end of my subsequent pregnancy, my OB was ready to just check me in and have me stay at the hospital until the baby came. We were all kind of shocked (myself included) when I decided to go home. Turns out the beeping machines just were not very welcoming. At thirty-seven weeks, I scheduled an appointment every day of the week, just to be put on the fetal monitor. (Christine)

A good care provider is usually happy to offer reassurance, so never feel like you cannot go in. Everybody is working together to help you move through these last weeks to a successful birth. Getting objective data to add to your own sense of your baby's well-being can go a long way toward providing the full picture.

> I went into the hospital because baby's movements changed. I'm thirty-four weeks tomorrow. I'm being seen twice a week, once with my OBGYN and the other with my MFM. I get a Doppler and in-depth umbilical cord monitoring every Friday. (Danielle)

One gift your previous baby may have given you is that you are the best advocate for yourself and your unborn baby. Nevertheless, getting what you need to cope with your anxiety can be exhausting. For example, Laurie's deceased baby's thirty-two-week ultrasound was on target for growth, but when she was born at forty-one-plus weeks, she weighed just over five pounds. In this current pregnancy, she wanted more growth scans and advocated strongly for this arrangement. Her doctor finally agreed to assess every three weeks starting at thirty-two weeks. At one point she noticed her baby having hiccups more than six times a day, a symptom she had learned may be associated with increased risk of stillbirth.[1] At her thirty-four-week appointment, the nurse told her this was "normal," that she should just relax and not be so anxious, but agreed to do a BPP. She learned her baby scored eight out of eight, and that is what she needed: reassurance.

> I already feel crazy, and when you need to explain issues and ask for more reassurance, it is exhausting. It's bad enough when your family says things, but my doctor is dismissing me too. (Laurie)

Don't let your anxiety stop you from calling. It is better to leave knowing more about your baby and get the reassurance that your baby is alive.

> I make more visits than I'm scheduled to make. Sunday I was feeling really nervous and I called the doctor on call and he didn't think that I really needed to go in and get checked. "Well, if they are hard contractions, if they are coming five minutes apart, then come in." He just said, "If everything's fine, they are just going to send you home." I was thinking, "Check me out, and send me home." I went in, everything was okay, and I felt better. (Joy)

It is common to have intermittent contractions, sometimes called Braxton Hicks, throughout pregnancy and more so in the last weeks as your body prepares for birth. When contractions are more frequent, longer, and stronger, this can be a sign of actual labor. Be sure and follow your MCP's plan when you think you might be in actual labor. If you are able to have rest periods during the day, it is important to lie on your side and stay hydrated. Just as you would pay attention to your baby's crying after birth, think about this time as "feeding your baby" during pregnancy. During these rest times, put your hands on your belly to feel the difference between the bumps and rolls of your baby's movements and the hardness of the uterus when it contacts. This process helps you learn the difference between the two. When you have contractions, communicate with your baby that this is what labor will feel like. Practice slow, even breathing, visualizing your baby rocking up and down with each breath. This can be a way to help calm yourself and your baby.

PREPARATIONS AT HOME
Preparing to bring your baby home is not something you can even imagine happening until you bring a living baby home. It is quite normal to get nothing ready, and this is very individual. You may remember the pain of taking everything down or just closing off the nursery. You may not want to change the room and just add things for it to be a little different, especially if you are having a different gender this time. Or you may do what one mother did: order the baby furniture and have note cards placed in the nursery room for her parents to have the room ready when they came home from the hospital.

> I didn't redecorate his room entirely. I just added on to the room. I took out his clothes; I saved some just for him. I bought a lot of neutral stuff; I just had Arrow [first child born after loss] wear it. And then some of the really boy things of Stone's [second baby boy] are here. (Danielle)

> We did move to a different home and did not bring her back to the same room that we would have brought Luke to. But we're still using the same bedding. I feel like we want to share that with her. (Kim)

You may also feel hopeful and will slowly start making small preparations at whatever comfort level feels right for you. Remember, all your baby really needs is your closeness, a place to sleep and to be held, fed, and changed.

I think it's still in our minds that something could go wrong, but there's been a lot of joy in the last month with the anticipation of her arrival. We had the birthing classes and we had the breastfeeding class. All this increases our preparation and our anticipation and excitement to have her with us. (Kim)

We were putting it off. Then Stacy, slowly, to celebrate each week that we got through, would buy one small thing. Now that we're at twenty-nine weeks, she's kind of letting herself kind of ease into it. (Russ)

In the end, if you can celebrate each day regardless of how frightened you are, try to embrace the time you have. You may also buy a few small things, giving yourself hope that all will be well.

I have come to the conclusion I need to love this baby, so if I only have six weeks or twelve weeks I will be able to say to this baby and to myself, I loved you to the fullest. We had our time together and I have no regrets. While I couldn't always do that every day, that was my optimism and hope. (Stacy)

BIRTH PREPARATION

Your past experience has a profound impact on how you will approach your upcoming birth. Because birth meant death, it can be hard to get yourself to a place where you can trust the birthing process. You may not have taken a birthing class before your previous baby was born and are aware you will not fit into a standard class. You may even be thinking of avoiding preparation, choosing instead to "plow through" labor and birth, determined not to think about the emotional impact this might have on you and your partner. A discussion around unexpected outcomes in a regular birthing class will have a different meaning for you.

We went to a regular all-day birthing class that said it would cover unexpected outcomes in the afternoon. Over lunch we discussed whether to share our previous losses. When the discussion began, the topic was "What if you have an unplanned caesarean or a boy when you really wanted a girl?" We looked at each other and decided not to share our history. (Adrienne)

In the past thirty years, special prenatal and birthing classes have been developed for families who have suffered a previous loss. These sessions take into account your previous experience and work with your anxieties. There are some online birthing classes specifically for families who have suffered a loss and childbirth instructors in private practice who can provide such a service.[2] You can ask for individual preparation from your health care provider or call the hospital where you will be giving birth to meet with someone to help you prepare. If you have no other option and decide to take a regular birthing class, let the instructor know ahead of time that you have had a previous loss.

> When we were filling out the questionnaire for this class, they ask you if you've had other pregnancies and if you have other children. We had to write still-born. We don't feel it's right to say *no* because we do have another child. Now granted, it's a lot different giving birth to a two-pound baby than an eight-pound baby, but I'm not worried about any of it. (Deanna)

Breastfeeding and infant care are standard topics in a birthing class for parents before the baby is born. But learning about breastfeeding can be difficult until you know this baby is safe. It is common to wait until your baby is in your arms before you can imagine the possibility of breastfeeding. From your viewpoint, this makes perfect sense.

> I can't imagine being a parent and taking that baby home with me. I try to visualize how our family is going to be when we are at home and have this little baby, just loving him and taking care of him. Sometimes you can't get past today, let alone look at bringing that baby home. (Susan)

You may also choose not to breastfeed or perhaps might not be able to emotionally "go there." Some women who have experienced past abuse are also unable to contemplate breastfeeding. You may want to know the amount of milk your baby is drinking, so you may wish to express breastmilk and use a bottle. You might not trust that your body is able to sustain a baby's life. Whatever the reason, feeding directly from the breast might not be for you. The important thing is to discuss what you want with your MCP so that you can receive the appropriate support.

TOURING BEFORE LABOR

It is important that you at least tour the area where you will be giving birth. You may feel you don't need a tour or want to go to the hospital, thinking,

"Why would I go there before I have to?" Touring the space with someone who knows your story before you are in active labor can help you minimize any painful memories that may surface in the environment. Touring can also help you process feelings you may not even know you carry. For instance, one couple, on entering the birthing room, saw the overbed table and had a flashback of seeing their deceased baby on the tray.

> You might see something; you'll remember something in the NICU; it will bring back all these memories, stuff that you have forgotten about. (John)

A "standard" hospital tour with other pregnant parents may not be the best choice for you. If you have no other option, tell the person giving you the tour that you have had a previous loss. During the tour, you may need time to revisit the environment, including the sights and smells, ask questions about the equipment, and discuss your anxiety and needs with the staff.

> For my husband, going to the labor room really helped him with some of his fears. He was really nervous while we were there but at least he had a perspective. It's a different labor room; it looks different even though the equipment is similar, the bed is similar, and he's beginning to feel more comfortable with it. It's not going to be a brand-new place for him. (Roxanne)

If you are birthing at the same hospital, you may want to avoid the room where your previous baby died and reflect that on your birth plan. However, some parents will want to be in the same space and find it healing.

> I went into the room where Brennan had been born and laid on that bed, just spending some time dealing with this [anxiety]. I cried, I relived it, I remembered as much as I could; I thought about his face, which was fading. I wrote him a poem: basically said we were going to have another baby, how much I missed him, and that I would always love him. The process of going from anxiety, to crying, to writing a poem, to reliving the experience, gave me so much calm and peace that I fell asleep. I woke up; I felt refreshed. (Sherokee)

Another couple chose a different room but went back into the room with their healthy newborn in their arms to look one last time at the room where their deceased baby had been born.

We decided that we could not be in the same room that we delivered in last time. We could not even bring ourselves to walk past the door of the room we delivered in. I know some families want to try and be in the same room, and if we are fortunate to have more children, we might want that next time. (Christine)

PACKING BAGS

Packing bags for use in hospital is likely to trigger memories for you from last time. Most parents will include a range of items that might not be considered "normal," like the plot number for the burial certificate or an outfit suitable for a coffin. However, even at this stage, you just don't dare think that everything will be okay. Bringing a photo or something that represents your deceased baby can also be an important part of your birthing experience. This helps you create a space where you can feel safe and be comfortable to give birth to your baby. It also is another reminder of those caring for you that this is not your first baby.

> People knew that Micah had died and made accommodations. They bent the rules for us on some things because of the importance of this baby to us. Like letting the doula do a video of the C-birth, letting me hold her for a long time when she was first born. They assigned me a postpartum room before surgery so that my doula could go in and set the room up how it would be: our space when I came out of recovery. (Cheryl)

Think about preparations for what you may want for yourself too! It's becoming more and more common for you to continue to wear your own comfortable loose-fitting clothes during labor and birth in hospital. This may be even more important for you because wearing a hospital gown may remind you of your loss.

Aware of what little time you had with your deceased baby, another way to prepare can be to consider writing a brief note to family members about your expectations after this baby is born.[3]

> I am writing the letter to our families as I am anticipating very heightened emotions. I think that getting some of my thoughts on paper ahead of time will help give us all the smoothest experience. I want to explain things while I am well rested and not overwhelmed with (hopefully) taking care of a newborn and also

tending to my grief. Babies can bring out the crazy in families, especially when it's a baby following a loss and all the extra-complicated emotions that come with it. I'm going to include specifics about how I may or may not be open to others holding this baby. I'm also going to prep them that having a new baby will bring up new levels of grief, and for them to not expect us to be just happy. (Amanda)

One father said he often wished he had not let everyone in the room hold his baby, who died unexpectedly the next day of a heart defect. He thought he had more time to hold his child. So in the new pregnancy he was very protective, making family understand that they might not get to hold the new baby for some time.

TIMING AND MODE OF GIVING BIRTH

When the optimal time is for giving birth is a multifaceted decision for both you and your care provider, and you may have already had this discussion earlier in your pregnancy with your MCP. Current medical care, especially in the United States, due to the "39-week rule," dictates there should be a medical reason for an induction. While the rule was established to prevent problems with newborn babies, this has made it more difficult for PAL parents. Timing of birth is not an easy decision to make, so you need a frank discussion with your care provider around the risks and benefits of being induced or waiting to have your baby naturally. If you already have had a successful pregnancy after your loss, you may still need to have this discussion. For example, Danielle's first subsequent baby was born at thirty-seven weeks because her blood pressure was increasing. Her MCP was treating her third pregnancy as "normal," which was concerning because her baby was measuring larger. She advocated for her second subsequent baby based on her history and knowledge of this situation:

> My current baby is measuring a week and a half bigger than his gestational age, and I know that Jude's weight may have been a cause for his death because he was so heavy. He probably pinched that part of the umbilical cord that was weak. Then I had another doctor, who did Jude's autopsy, who also said that the ratio of his weight to my placenta was smaller. He was big, and that makes me fear that my unborn baby is already big now so there could be problems. I want to get him out early. (Danielle)

You may intuitively know that your baby needs to be born by caesarean. From the beginning of her pregnancy, one mother asked for a caesarean birth because of the cord insertion problem in her previous pregnancy. In spite of testing done twice a week, her previous son died suddenly at just over thirty-eight weeks. She had changed doctors to one who agreed to a caesarean at thirty-seven weeks, weighing the risks against the benefits. Depending on why your previous baby died, you may have to negotiate what is best for you.

> Jolene was born with a cord around her neck and a true knot in her cord. I don't want to imagine what could have happened if I wouldn't have had my C-section. I'm glad that my doctor and I agreed on C-section. It's really important to follow mother's instinct. Jolene was almost three days in NICU due to water in her lungs. (Michaela)

You or your unborn baby may have medical conditions that play into the decision (e.g., placenta previa or high blood pressure, small-for-dates baby, or breech position). Your emotional well-being can also play into timing and mode of birth. Safety for you and your baby is everyone's goal. A frank discussion with your health care provider is key to creating the best birth option for you and your baby.

> The birth plan was to induce the baby two weeks before her due date because my stillborn daughter had gone four days over when she died. I wasn't going to go anywhere near my due date. (Lydia)

> I had an exhausting day with an NST at the hospital: discussion of induction, lots of emotions about such burdensome decisions! The doctor didn't check my cervix, though he checked for amniotic fluid as I thought I might be leaking fluid this morning. I've been telling the baby to get things going. (Michelle)

You may decide, with your MCP, that birthing by caesarean is the best option for you. You may have an issue in your pregnancy that could be managed by having a caesarean as a choice.

> It was a little glitch when we discovered she was breech and we had to have the C-section because we were looking forward to having a vaginal birth. They did try an external version, but it didn't work and it was rather painful. (Jonathan)

As much as possible, try to carry hope that all will be well. As you prepare to release this baby into the world, it may be helpful to find someone to walk you through the guided imagery from chapter 6. You may also choose to record yourself reading this and listen back to help you feel less anxious.

BIRTH PLANS

In your previous birth, you may have been like many other parents who wrote a "birth plan" of what you would or would not want, such as walking during labor, no medications, or an epidural at some point in labor. Now all you want is a baby who is alive.

> With Jude I did a plan: no machines, no monitors. Then afterwards I thought, "Oh, you were such a fool. Your birth plan should be 'I just want a live baby.'" (Danielle)

Writing a birth plan can be very helpful. You may have the same doctor caring for you but not have the same health care team. Even though your history will be in your medical records, you want the providers caring for you to know your history in your own words. This does not have to be long or complicated—perhaps "Our baby died eighteen months ago and it feels like it happened yesterday. We will need much support in this labor and birth experience." Recognize, however, that no matter what your situation, any plan can take a detour, and that is okay. You can change your mind and adapt your plan as you go along.

> We would have preferred if everyone who entered our room knew our history before walking through the door. As much as we tried to communicate to our nurses to tell the staff, someone would walk in and ask me if this was my first baby. In between contractions, I would respond, no, my first baby died. Just as the nurses hung a white silk rose on my door when Madison died, a sign on the door in both my L&D and maternity rooms would have made things a little easier. Perhaps a sign in the shape of a rainbow, signifying hope after a storm [the previous loss], would be appropriate. (Christine)

You can also put a sign outside your door, as one mother did, that lets everyone in the room know you have had a previous loss.

R A I N B O W

BIRTH

IN

PROGRESS

PROVIDERS, PLEASE READ

Please be kind, patient, and respectful. Help us have a positive birthing experience.

Our first birthing experience was very sad and traumatic as we knew we wouldn't be bringing our baby home after anxiously anticipating his arrival for 40 weeks. This pregnancy has been a long, hard journey and we are experiencing a variety of emotions from fear to excitement.

How you can help:

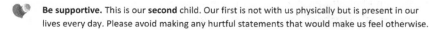 **Be supportive.** This is our **second** child. Our first is not with us physically but is present in our lives every day. Please avoid making any hurtful statements that would make us feel otherwise.

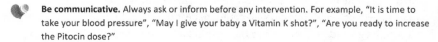 **Be communicative.** Always ask or inform before any intervention. For example, "It is time to take your blood pressure", "May I give your baby a Vitamin K shot?", "Are you ready to increase the Pitocin dose?"

Be empathetic. It is never too late to say "I'm sorry".

Thank you for your support!

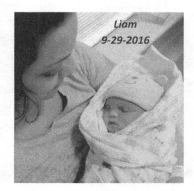

Liam
9-29-2016

Courtesy of Anna Calix

THE LAST DAYS

Even as you work to keep your anxiety at a level you can cope with, it is okay to ask for what you need to get to the end of your pregnancy. This may mean asking your doctor to admit you to hospital, especially if you live outside a large metropolitan area and are worried about getting stuck in traffic even going to your appointments. For another mother, overwhelmed with anxiety due to eleven previous losses (two late losses), it made sense for her MCP to help with her anxiety in the last week of pregnancy by just admitting her to the hospital during her last days of pregnancy. Again, this is very individual, would not be offered routinely, but might be something you could negotiate.

> I made it to thirty-six weeks four days. My anxiety that day couldn't be controlled; I even had a massage that evening to try and relax. The baby didn't move once throughout the massage, so I spent the massage a hot mess of worry. As soon as the massage was over, I pulled out the Doppler, and all was fine—except not for me emotionally. I went home and broke down. I couldn't spend one night more worrying and checking. I was admitted to the hospital for constant monitoring. My doctor came in the morning to check in on me, and I started bawling. I felt like I had let everyone down. I was trying to be so strong and hold it together and not inconvenience anyone. And then she said something that made all those feelings go away. She said, "Honey, I'm surprised you didn't come in earlier." She wasn't being critical. She was telling me that she couldn't believe—with my story—I could make it this long. I felt so relieved and ready to let go and let everyone in the hospital take care of me. I spent the next four days sleeping. They had me hooked up to the monitor and I didn't have to worry about a thing. They kept a watchful eye as I let my body surrender. My body rested both mentally and physically. When thirty-seven weeks came, we started the process of induction. (Kari)

You may have times of grieving more intensely as you approach birth, remembering the unexpected memories of the last weeks of your deceased baby's life. This is not uncommon and can be expected as you prepare to meet this new baby.

> Grief has come back with a stronger force than the past few months. It's just really hard for me to talk about Jude and not just sob and start to think that this baby may die, too. I'm hanging in there, though. (Danielle)

> I was having flashbacks of the days when he died. (Michaela)

Two weeks before her son's birth, waking up at night unable to sleep, missing her previous baby, and longing to hold this new baby in her arms, one mother put her feelings into verse:

At Last This Baby and This Mother

Hello baby, I'm glad you're here.

Listen to my words, follow my lead, I have wonderful things to teach you.

Be strong baby. Bear the burden of my

doubts and fears. They will lessen as we grow.

I'm ready to hold you close, to swallow the

scent of your tiny head, to sing you songs about the moon and stars

At last baby, enter this cold and crazy world.

We'll share our strength and courage and watch each other grow. I love you.

Hello Mom. I'm glad you are listening to me.

I don't mind that you are afraid. I can help you with that.

I'm soon to be evicted from this warm and

precious womb. I need help. Your world is a cold and crazy place.

I'm ready to feel your fingers against my

skin. Hold me close, sing me songs.

At last Mom, listen to my heart, follow my

lead. For I have wonderful things to teach you. I love you.

(Used with permission from Mona McNeely)

THE BIRTH DAY

Even if you have toured the place where you will give birth and believe you are well prepared, be aware that you and your partner will have strong feelings, especially during the pushing stage. Be sure this is reflected on your birth plan, and remind your care providers that both of you will need more support.

When I was pushing, I didn't want to push. I was afraid I would see another dead baby. (Ann)

It can be helpful to know that in labor your baby will also be working with you during each contraction, pushing his/her body to move down into the birth canal. This visualization can be a positive message for your partner to remind you of during contractions.

You may be doing fine and suddenly be surprised that unexpected feelings can occur. One mother was unprepared for her grief to surface as she began to birth her healthy daughter.

At the delivery, that's when I started thinking about the losses again and was almost shocked. I'm starting to push and it's like just dawning on me, this baby is actually going to be here and nothing bad is going to happen. I started grieving all over again for the two losses. This is the time these two pregnancies are coming back to me? But tears were rolling down my face during pushing. I was kind of in my own little world. I didn't tell anybody: "Gee, you guys, I'm thinking about the losses." I just kind of shut down because when I pushed I was just kind of focused anyway. I shut my eyes. Here comes this baby and I'm so happy, but I'm sad because I lost these other two little babies. (Marybeth)

In labor everybody is focused on the mother, so you may also consider hiring a doula to support both you and your partner. This is a person trained to assist you as a couple during childbirth and who can also provide support to your family after the baby is born. Today there are doulas who have had special training in working with bereaved parents.[4]

After Madison, I was certain that I needed a doula. I needed someone to be an additional advocate for me in the hospital, as well as someone who had experience and could help me through L&D—not just the physical aspects but also the emotional ones. I had a doula for my subsequent pregnancies who was a nurse, but also very holistic. She had me listen to this *Calm Birth* CD during my pregnancies. It's now online in MP3 format.[5] I also really liked that I could call my doula any time before labor to ask any questions. Essentially, she was someone I could go to as an additional resource to my OB office if I was nervous about the baby's movement, or anything else. She made two home visits before I delivered and went over exercises that I could do to help prepare for labor (cat/cow position, etc.). One time she came and just walked with me to make sure I was moving enough. We also just talked about my worries and my preferences (one of which was that no one ask me if this was my first pregnancy). She was a wonderful resource for us and understood (as best she could) how difficult the loss was and how much support I would need in the subsequent pregnancies. After Harry's delivery, she was someone I could talk to about the mixed emotions I had after his birth and my trouble bonding with him. My husband thought she was essential to us. (Christine)

THE BORN ALIVE BABY

Even after reassurance throughout your pregnancy that all is well with your baby, it is not until the baby is safely in your arms or you hear your baby cry that you will truly believe you have made it. Or until the Apgar scores are known.[6] Or until you get your living baby home. Delivery of a healthy baby may not assuage ALL of your concerns right away, and that is okay.

> They put him on my chest, and I whispered to Derek, "He's alive." There was nothing in this pregnancy that would have given us any thought otherwise, but it was just that realization that "Hey, we made it." He's here, he's okay; we can see him and hold him and know that he's all right. (Carissa)

You will experience bittersweet emotions when seeing your new baby. An unanticipated new layer of grief is common. In your overwhelming joy, holding this healthy baby, you now understand more deeply what you missed with the death of your previous baby.[7]

> I think it made us even sadder for the loss of our daughter because we didn't really know what we didn't have until we had something else. Then it just felt empty. (Roxanne)

Be aware that your new baby may also look just like your deceased baby, even if the genders are different. Remember, this is a sibling, so of course he or she will look familiar.

Family and friends may notice this as well and may not know what to say. Don't be afraid to initiate this conversation. It is really common with living siblings and reminds people that there is still a missing person in your family.

I had another daughter, and ironic circumstances duplicated my first daughter. (Melba)

SUMMARY

This chapter has addressed the last weeks of pregnancy and your upcoming birth. As you move closer to birth, do as much as you can to relieve your anxiety. Try to celebrate that you have done hard work to get yourself and this baby to this point. Your awareness of this new unborn baby and consistent testing from your health care team can help give you reassurance that your baby is safe.

REFLECTIONS

- Are there any leftover questions that you still need to discuss with your MCP?
- Do you feel you have prepared family and friends for what you might need from them around your birth?
- Take time to connect with the unborn baby, remembering that you are doing this birth together.
- Remembering your last weeks with your deceased baby, try to reflect on your continued love as you greet the new little sibling.

8

Beautiful Babies Breathing

After the birth of your baby, even as you celebrate the birth, you begin a different journey: parenting this new little one while not forgetting your deceased baby. This chapter will cover the many feelings you might encounter coming to terms with your new baby as a separate little person whose growth and development is a constant reminder of what you have missed with your other child.

> This journey is just about as difficult to navigate as loss and PAL [pregnancy after loss], but not quite as hard because our babies are here! (Anna)

EARLY DAYS

Anticipating what the early days will be like can be confusing. Every day of your pregnancy was focused on protecting your new baby while grieving the loss of your deceased baby. It can be hard to believe you have made it with a living baby. It is important to know that all parents early postpartum have many physical and emotional ups and downs, even with older, healthy children. Yours will be more intense, with mixed bittersweet emotions. This baby is a powerful reminder of your other baby's birth and death.

> The whole pregnancy I felt like I was even more focused on Tino than Lucian, even though I was very worried about Lucian, of course, the whole way through. (Karen)

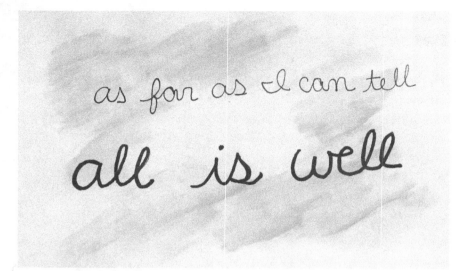

as far as I can tell

all is well

Courtesy of Diana Le-Cabrera

I feel guilty because the grief is still there, this push and pull of missing her. (Laurie)

If you birthed in the hospital, you may want to have a sign of some kind on your door to remind the staff that this is not your first baby.

ADMISSION TO NURSERY

You may have unexpectedly had your baby early or had complications where your newborn needed to go to a special care nursery or newborn intensive care unit. You will have to emotionally readjust as the medical team takes over your baby's care. While you are immensely grateful this care is available for your baby, you are unsure of your role, bringing back memories of your previous baby's death. You may have a flashback to your previous baby, so let the staff know your history.

I was amazed, being put in that mode, how much the smells in the special care nurseries brought that all back because Bailey [deceased baby] was in the spe-

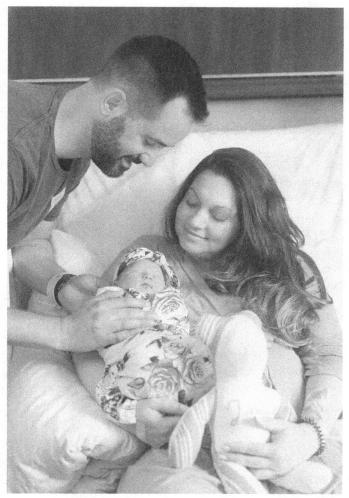

Courtesy of Danielle Ondarza

cial care for ten days. And Max [subsequent baby] was in for seven days because of the IV antibiotics for his respiratory infection. (Ann)

Even if your baby is in an isolette around noisy equipment, your baby knows your voice and will react to your presence. Talk to your baby; gently touching and giving reassurance is important for both of you. Going home without your baby also brings memories of leaving the hospital the last time without your deceased baby. If possible, negotiate with staff to stay with your baby.

> She was in the hospital after she was born with bilirubin (jaundice) for three days under the lights [phototherapy]. They had us take her home first and just keep her in the sun. We were supposed to bring her in every two days to get her bilirubin checked. It went up to seventeen, so they ended up admitting her. They wanted me to go home but I wouldn't go. (Diane)

You may have unexpectedly learned that your baby has a health issue that needs to be taken care of at a later date. While grateful it was found, it can also be hard to wait, and, like this mother, you may have to change your maternity leave plans if your baby has medical issues:

> They were checking her to go home when they did an ultrasound and found the coarctation, which is a narrowing of the aorta. What usually happens is people don't find those and the baby goes home, and the reason they find them is the baby gets really sick a week later. My whole maternity leave was kind of hard because she was getting skinny and we had to wait to see if we were going to have the surgery or not. Once we had the surgery everything was fine. (Ann)

YOUR NEW BABY

The gender of your baby may also be something that you are dealing with. You may accidentally call your new baby by your deceased baby's name. This is common for every parent with other children. Your babies are siblings, so there may be a family likeness between your children. It may take time for you to get to know this baby as a separate individual. Confusion over gender can happen after having a second subsequent baby as well, something you may have to process with your partner.

> It was easier to separate Jackson [first son after loss] from Madison because he was a boy. Harry was a struggle [second son]. I couldn't seem to separate him from Jackson, and that seemed to impact my ability to bond with him. Over time, Harry's differences and his unique personality have become clearer, so that has helped immensely, but it was very difficult for me during the first two weeks after his birth. (Christine)

Now that Emma is here, the girls are completely separate in my mind. Even though she wears the clothes and bows we bought for Lily, plays with the toys, even sleeps in the bassinet, I know and feel in my heart that she is a completely different baby. It sounds strange. Of course they are different babies, but a grieving heart can do strange things to your mind. I think part of the separation comes from the fact that Emma is so full of life: her smile, her laugh, her little coos. My memories of Lily are only of death. My still, silent baby girl. When I held her, she was cold. Every time I pick Emma up, I soak in her warmth. (Lauren)

VISITORS

Your family and friends may be very keen to visit and may not understand or even take offense to you wanting to keep visitors to a minimum while you are all getting to know your new baby. Also, you are probably not the only one having mixed feelings about the new baby's arrival. Family and friends may also be struggling with mixed emotions and want to see your living baby to reassure themselves that all is well. They may also be revisiting emotions from last time.

ANNOUNCING THE BIRTH

Now more than ever your deceased baby may not be mentioned by others. They may all think that you have now gotten on with your lives and no longer think or need to talk about your baby who died. Instead, your new baby is an everyday reminder of the deceased baby you once held. One way to help with this issue, which has become more common today, is to include your deceased baby in a birth announcement. This reminds others that your baby is still an important member of your family. Some parents do not include their deceased baby's name because they feel that it does not belong there. It is completely up to you and a very personal decision.

NORMAL NEWBORN DEVELOPMENT

The first month of life is a time of upheaval for all parents, even if you had older living children. Added to the normal ups and downs, you have different challenges that may make you feel overwhelmed, more emotional and anxious. Unless your deceased baby lived for a short time, you probably never saw your baby with open eyes. This baby will be different. Right from birth

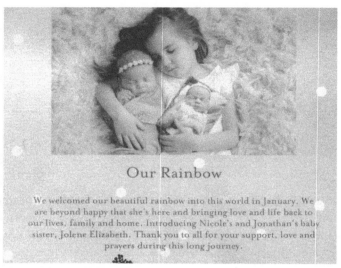

Our Rainbow

We welcomed our beautiful rainbow into this world in January. We are beyond happy that she's here and bringing love and life back to our lives, family and home. Introducing Nicole's and Jonathan's baby sister, Jolene Elizabeth. Thank you to all for your support, love and prayers during this long journey.

Courtesy of Michaela Backiel

babies open their eyes and can see a distance of about twelve inches and, in an alert state, will gaze at you with open eyes and wonder, just as anxious to know what you look like, too! If you place your face on either side of your baby's ears, he will turn to your voice. This will be a very magical moment for you.

As you adjust from a very stressful pregnancy, your baby is adjusting to the outside world. You may not trust that all is well, wondering: What is normal newborn development? How do I know whether my baby is healthy? Request that your health care providers do the newborn exams in front of you, explaining what they are seeing. This will give you an opportunity to share concerns and ask questions.

Babies naturally have extra fluid when born, so it is common for all newborns to initially lose weight, but this loss of weight can alarm you. It is also normal for a newborn baby's skin to be a little yellow (jaundiced). This usually peaks around day four or five and is most often related to babies getting rid of the extra red blood cells they don't need anymore. However, there are occasionally other health-related reasons for jaundice, so be sure and check with your pediatrician to be reassured your baby's weight loss and jaundice level is in the normal range.

FEEDING

Feeding your baby can be challenging after a loss. Remember, your baby has never felt hunger before and now has to figure out when he or she may be hungry or full and what to do with gas. Is he or she gaining enough weight? For many bereaved parents, the issues in deciding how to feed their baby are quite different from those who have not experienced the death of a baby. You may not have taken a breastfeeding class before birth, thinking, "Why would I take a class on feeding a baby whom I don't believe will really come home?" You might not have had the chance to breastfeed your last baby and remember that you really wanted to.

> Flynn was in the special care nursery for two weeks, which made breastfeeding very difficult. That didn't help after the loss of his brother, who I didn't get to feed at all. (Skye)

Breastfeeding can be challenging for all new moms. It is rarely like the pictures you see in magazines. Don't let those around you say that you should supplement if you don't want to. The more you breastfeed, the more milk you will make. Your baby may want to feed within an hour or so after feeding, and you may think you are losing your milk supply. But in actuality, your baby is nursing to help increase your milk supply. Cluster feeding is quite normal for all babies.[1] You can also feel that you don't trust your body to nourish this baby. Fortunately, this mother got support from her parenting after loss group and did not supplement, realizing he needed to cluster feed:

> I went to my postpartum visit and he hadn't gained enough weight so the doctor told me to start bottles. I was devastated. I couldn't keep my first baby alive in my body and now I couldn't keep his brother alive with my breastfeeding. (Caroline)

If you're concerned about your baby not gaining weight, you need a plan. Sometimes it's a feeding issue or medical issue, and some babies are just slow gainers. Do not wait to contact a breastfeeding consultant if you find breastfeeding painful, especially discomfort in your breasts or nipples. Extreme pain that continues during the entire feeding should be reported. A peer-support breastfeeding counselor or lactation consultant can usually assist.

Breastfeeding is actually a challenge. I keep having different types of problems. We're working on the problems one by one. He had a tongue tie, which affected his ability to latch correctly, we had taken care of, then it grew back, and we had to do it again. But he's growing well, and it's definitely improved this last month. (Karen)

Jackson didn't gain weight very quickly. At the two-week checkup he was at the same weight he was when he left the hospital. So there was "Should we go to formula?" "Is there a problem with my supply?" We saw a lactation consultant, and we finally figured out I had to do some breast compression [expression] to help him get the milk. Then he started gaining within a few days, but it was nerve-racking for us. (Christine)

You may choose to feed your baby into toddlerhood in order to compensate for not being able to feed your deceased baby, as this mother found:

Breastfeeding both my rainbow babies into their toddler years was a way for me to take in every part of them. It was more than simply feeding them. It felt like a way for me to practice gratitude that they were born alive and that I was being fully present with them. (Kari)

Is formula feeding okay? You may feel conflicted and feel guilt that you have chosen not to breastfeed. If you recall the pain associated with full breasts and no baby to give the milk to, you may elect to bottle feed right from the start to avoid that painful reminder. If you had expressed (pumped) for your sick, premature baby who died, you might decide it is all too difficult to try again, particularly if your next baby is also born prematurely. Feeding your baby either by breast or by bottle is a personal choice.

CALMING YOUR BABY

Your baby's cry is a very powerful form of communication, your baby's way of calling for help. Placing your hand on your baby's chest, or helping your baby keep his or her arms and legs tucked in, gives him or her a sense of security by mimicking the boundary of the uterine wall before birth. A baby whose hands are wrapped in a blanket or whose T-shirt has mittens extending over his or her hands and fingers is unable to help comfort and calm himself or herself. Position your baby's hands close to his face. Sucking on his hands

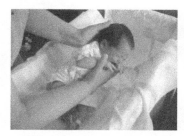

Start with your baby on his back.
Be sure clothing does not cover baby's hands.
Use one hand to hold the baby's hands
to his mouth.

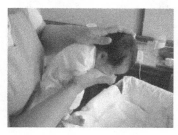

Gently roll baby over so he is facing downward.
Bring baby up to your chest
with baby facing outward.
Allow baby's body to flex forward,
keeping baby's hands in contact with his mouth.
He may begin to suckle on his fingers.

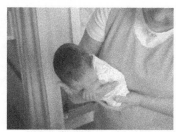

Use your other hand to help baby flex his legs.
You may sway from side to side or bounce gently.

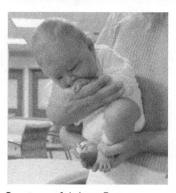

Feeling calm and secure in the flex hold.

Courtesy of Jolene Pearson

can help your baby feel calmer and more secure. You might have noticed this tendency during an ultrasound. If you have tried a number of things, such as burping, feeding, changing, rocking, and holding, and your baby continues to cry, then try placing your baby in the flex-hold position (see page 97). This position takes your baby back to being in the womb, rocking up and down with each breath you took during pregnancy.

Responding to your newborn's cries is not spoiling. It teaches your baby to ask for and receive help. You may also want to hear your baby's cry because you didn't hear your other baby's.

> I let her cry briefly before I go to her because it assures me she is still alive. (Jen)

You may have a baby who is difficult to calm, which can be very distressing after months of anticipating all would be well once your baby was born. Crying means your baby is distressed. Reach out to your pediatrician to help assess what might be going on. Never hesitate to confide in your partner, your friends, your family, or others if your feelings are overwhelming.

SLEEP

A common question all new parents ask is: How do I help him or her learn to sleep? Sleep issues can be more of a challenge for you than the baby.

> So besides eating for the first month or so, sleeping was a real struggle for us. The problem was he was still getting up every two hours and we were both working and exhausted. (Sid)

You may be overly concerned about checking on your baby and not being able to get a good night's rest. After the loss of a baby, it will take time to learn to trust that your baby will stay alive while sleeping.

> I remember watching her at night quite intently to make sure she was breathing. I had her in the crib right by the bed. (Betty)

You may need your baby near you or have your baby in another room with a monitor for reassurance that all is well. You and your partner may take turns being up with the baby or take turns sleeping in the same room as your baby. If you have grandparents staying over, they can help with care, giving them a chance to get to know the baby, too. Discuss with your partner what will work for you.

UNDERSTANDING YOUR BABY'S SLEEP PATTERNS

Understanding the two patterns of newborn sleep is helpful. All babies have patterns of sleep, from a deep sleep to light sleep. Your baby needs deep sleep in order to grow and develop. When in deep sleep, your baby's body is very still, and breathing is slow and even. It is sometimes hard to detect a baby's breathing in a deep sleep: your baby may startle but quickly return to sleep. Seeing your baby in a deep sleep can remind you of your deceased baby. You may want to put your hand on your baby's chest to feel the up and down movements for reassurance. This is particularly true if comments were made about your deceased baby—for example, "He just looks like he is asleep." This situation is common and will gradually pass.

> When Flynn is sleeping he looks so much like his brother that I go in and check him more often. (Skye)

> One of my neuroses was when we put him down to sleep, I'd look at the time and think, "Okay, Jackson's still alive at eleven at night." Then I would go do whatever, and we'd check on him, and I'd be like, "He's still alive at four in the morning." I did this for about a month, and then it slowly faded away. (Christine)

Your baby will sometimes be in a light sleep, stretching or moving about. If you watch your baby's breathing, it will be more noticeable—your baby's eyes may move under their eyelids. In light sleep your baby will be more responsive to sound and movements and can be more easily awakened for a feeding. If you are trying to wake your baby for a feeding, look for light sleep, pick your baby up, and place your baby into a more upright position. The upright position and your voice are very effective ways to help your baby awaken for a feeding. Building your confidence for what is normal for your baby takes time. Your reassurance will come as you watch your baby's growth and development emerge.

SIDS

The fear of SIDS, and any other possible thing that could go wrong, is ever present. I remember looking at the clock every time I put Jackson down to sleep, and thinking, "Well, he's still alive right now." (Christine)

I talked with my husband last night about fearing Inzio would die and when it would happen. He said he had the same fears. (Brittany)

Back sleeping is the safest position for your baby and provides the best protection against sudden infant death syndrome (SIDS). You may worry that if your baby is back sleeping, he may spit up or vomit while asleep. Because babies automatically swallow or cough up such fluids, physiologists have shown NO increase in choking or other problems with babies sleeping on their backs. Millions of babies around the world sleep safely on their backs, and it is safe for your baby, too. It is also recommended to keep your baby's sleep area free of blankets and toys. If the weather is cool, you can dress your baby in a blanket sleeper for warmth; don't cover the baby with blankets. If keeping the baby close is what you need to do, it is important to follow the SIDS research-based guidelines. To reduce the risk of SIDS, the International Society for the Study and Prevention of Perinatal and Infant Death has several recommendations (listed in the references).[2]

Some parents choose to buy a baby monitor or sleep suit that sounds an alarm if it detects a drop in heart rate or movement. Other such monitors sound an alarm if the first two fall out of range. You may decide to purchase something similar or purchase sleep suits that monitor your baby's breathing. Using this kind of technology may allow you to sleep yourself. Any reputable baby store will have someone who will be able to assist in meeting your needs. However, such monitors can increase anxiety and interfere with sleep due to false alarms, so it can be a double-edged sword. Decide together what will work for you.

TALKING/COUNSELING

All new parents experience some emotional upheaval as they adjust to their new baby. Sleep deprivation and the intensity of caring for a newborn, especially after a loss, can impact your mental health. If your feelings are interfering with daily life, you will need to be seen. Never hesitate to get help beyond your family and friends to work through issues with a counselor or other trained professional. This makes feelings that are unconscious conscious, putting your thoughts in a different part of your brain, to examine. In fact, you may be ready to see a counselor now that you are safely through the pregnancy.

> My feeling is that loss moms are at a higher risk for PPD even after a live birth. As one mom I know put it: "I didn't realize that having a normal outcome would be so triggering." (Christine)

Never forget your baby has been an equal partner in this journey and felt your profound grief at the loss of your deceased baby. Don't be afraid to share your feelings and grief over the missing sibling; your baby listens and learns. Loving and enjoying this new baby does not take away your love for your deceased baby. You are giving reassurance that your baby is loved and wanted. You have enough love for all your children.

> While there is joy of the new baby's arrival, there is also deep sadness of all the milestones that the baby that died missed out on. (Christine)

> Tony's [live] birth didn't change who we were. It's not like he replaced anybody. It didn't change any of the past. (Mona)

SUMMARY

Family and friends may not understand why you are still sad. The early days will be more challenging because you have just been through a stressful pregnancy in which you were constantly on high alert to keep your baby safe. Don't be surprised that you will continue to cry at different times. Keep connected with other bereaved parents in your community or join an online support group for parenting after a loss.[3] They will be able to reassure you that it is still normal to feel sad and this new baby cannot and will not take away the memory of your baby who died. You are a parent to all your children, living and deceased.

9

The Male Perspective

This chapter focuses on your role as father/partner in this new pregnancy. Just as you may have grieved differently than your partner at the time of your previous loss, so will you face similar but different challenges now. You will need to cope with your own fears and anxieties while supporting your pregnant partner as you begin the emotional journey to welcome a new baby into the family.

FATHERS: YOU NEED RECOGNITION TOO

The role of the non-pregnant partner is often ignored or downplayed during pregnancy. How often have you heard "How is your wife/partner doing?" At the time of your loss the focus was on helping your partner get through the physical experience of the birth, causing your emotional state to be secondary. Yet you witnessed the trauma of watching your baby's birth, feeling helpless, unable to help your partner or save your deceased baby.

You may have felt or even been told the expectation for you was to be strong for your partner, deal with your grief, and go back to work to financially support your family. Friends and family may also have minimized your grief in this way. One mother learned why her husband didn't share many feelings with her:

> At Thanksgiving this year I heard that my mother-in-law told my husband when he called to say our baby died to "be strong for Skye." The message she gave him was "hold back your own grief." (Skye)

This message about what your role should be can follow into this new pregnancy. Others may continue to minimize that you have also suffered the loss of your baby and that you might be just as scared as your partner. You are on this journey, too, and, like your partner, know there are no guarantees of a healthy outcome.

> A pregnancy is not a one-person experience. The father's pain is intangible but it's acute nonetheless. I haven't been inside her body, but I think the father's feelings have been downplayed, ignored. Acknowledge their [fathers'] pain. They can be stoic on the outside, but unless they're just insensitive, at some level, unless it's an unwanted pregnancy, your pain is real. You're both going through this together. (Jeff)

> My own needs were the hardest thing to deal with at the time of loss and in our subsequent pregnancies because there is a balance between wanting recognition but also being afraid of taking some of that recognition away from your wife. (Darrell)

MOVING FORWARD

When thinking about how to move forward you may have had different questions than your partner in considering trying to get pregnant again. Often it is your partner who may be ready to move forward sooner because of the physical connection she had with your deceased baby. She feels the emptiness in her body and arms aching to hold her baby.

You also need to consider your finances. Will both of you be able to take time off from work again? If your previous baby was conceived via reproductive medicine, the expense of trying again can be costly. As a couple, are you both of like mind to risk trying again?

Another factor you may consider is whether the previous pregnancy was high risk due to the health of your partner or the baby. You may have not only lost your baby but also seen your partner near death in an intensive care unit. This experience can cause you to be cautious in even thinking about another pregnancy.

> I was pretty dead set against it. A fear-based decision is never usually the best one. I tried to make it from a loving base but it was hard. I mean, in a perfect world, if I could have another kid, then sure, I would have another kid. It's all

the "what if's" now that didn't exist before that kind of weigh you down. But the bigger thing I think was that I was just scared to lose my wife because it was scary seeing her that way. I don't really want to go through that again. (Bob)

Are the reasons for wanting another baby still valid? If you have older children, they can be your incentive for trying again. You want them to have a sibling, and they have already shown you that all pregnancies do not end in loss.

As odd as this may sound, I think Eliza was the determining factor of why we got pregnant again so quickly. That little buddy, the joy that she is. When we told her that we had lost the twins, she sat in the chair beside us looking out the window. Brittany asked her if she was okay, and she started bawling her eyes out: "I just want to be a big sister." So after about a month or two, we decided we wanted to give it a try again because we wanted her to be the big sister she wants to be. It was about two months later that we ended up conceiving. (Joe)

THE NEW PREGNANCY

You can have a range of different feelings when finding out you are going to be a father again. You may be excited but spend the first weeks not wanting to say too much, carrying feelings of happiness but protecting yourself from too much excitement, remembering the pain involved with the last experience. Can you face a period of emotional helplessness? Will you be able to cope with another loss? It's not that you don't want this baby—you want both babies.

I am excited because now I know that this is a new pregnancy. Maybe we can start all over. Maybe things can be normal from day one. But you still set up barriers where at any given time you're trying to prepare yourself for the worst. Because last time he did die, and you did start blazing your own trail for the grieving process. You always have the thought of a good outcome. You have hope and you want to think positive. (Len)

Before your baby died, you probably had no understanding that babies could die. Now you can't make any assumptions that any pregnancy will turn out okay. Particularly if you attended an infant loss support group, you may have learned all the other ways babies can die.

The more that you get involved in this whole pregnancy loss world, the more people you meet, and the more stories you hear, the more you're aware of all of the things that can happen—the miscarriages—nobody has answers. Loads of people have losses. (Mick)

You may have done early chromosomal testing to determine whether this new baby has any genetic risk factors, but you will still worry even if these test results are negative. To protect yourself, you may hold back feelings of hope until your unborn baby is further into the pregnancy.

We had genetic testing done, so I thought, "This will answer all our questions right away." The further along we get the better we feel, but it seems like nothing was wrong until the end with Lincoln, so we still don't really know. I think that's the biggest thing—you don't ever really know. It could all go sideways again. (Bob)

You may think your fears will go away when you pass the week when your previous loss occurred, and for some this does happen.

Probably in the back of our minds was that this could happen again until we got to that magic number, I guess, of eighteen weeks [the time of their previous loss]. That was kind of like, phew. And then getting past the date where he was born. (Mick)

However, this may not be the case for you. Continuing to worry is common and may be a part of your new pregnancy. Seeing your partner's number on your cell phone can be a trigger throughout the pregnancy.

I remember when Marci was pregnant with Noah, each time the phone rang and I was working, I would go, "Oh my goodness. Is this the call that will tell me that there is a problem?" Now Marci, having the baby inside her, wouldn't have that anxiety. She had her own anxiety. But living on pins and needles, that's something different for a father. (Jeff)

I noticed I had missed a call, so I checked it. She was on her way to the hospital; she thought there was something wrong again. That reminded me of the drive from the golf course to the emergency room last time. That was the most anxiety-ridden spell, or whatever, I've ever had in my life. I can't believe that this can happen again. And then I tried to convince myself that everything was going to be okay. Fortunately, it was. (Garrett)

If this is a concern for you, it can be helpful to ask her, when she calls, to first say, "Everything's fine. I just wanted you to know . . ."

TELLING OTHERS

Pregnancy itself is an incredibly intimate experience. One that follows the loss of a baby can leave you feeling vulnerable. You may hold back on telling others until later in the pregnancy or until your partner is obviously showing that she is pregnant and you feel you have no choice in sharing the news.

We didn't tell anyone until we were twenty-two weeks, not even our parents. I never was afraid to become attached. We just were real careful, just wanted to make sure that no one else got attached before we knew it was an okay deal. That's why we waited until twenty-two weeks to tell anyone. (Pete)

Knowing this will feel like a long pregnancy, you may take on a loving, protective role when dealing with family and friends in sharing the news. As a couple, you decide how much information you want to share and when to share with others.

I told my relatives, Ann's pregnant. Oh, congratulations, da da da. And I'm like, well, thank you, but . . . . Well, what's wrong? A lot of people just don't seem to understand, and I understand they don't understand. It's hard for me to fulfill their wishes of me being the happy new father when I feel like, well, something could happen, you know. It's a miracle that these kids come out with ten fingers and ten toes. (Kyle)

You may even wish you could just wait until your new baby is born! Sharing timelines that you chose can help as you approach the end of the pregnancy, so people aren't calling all the time asking how things are going. Some parents choose to be less candid and change the due date to two or three weeks later.

YOUR WORK AND WORK COLLEAGUES

When a baby dies, it is usually the father who goes back to work sooner than the mother. Your partner may need time to physically recover, but as one dad said, "The bills keep coming." This can cause you to postpone your grief even into a subsequent pregnancy, while also fearing another loss.

The death of your baby has changed who you are as a person. This is often not understood by others in your workplace, who may treat you like it is just any other workday.

> He went back to work right away after our loss, took two weeks off, which really wasn't enough. He'll refer to that time when some things were happening at work and his manager got angry with him about something and he said, "That was the week my baby died." He still can't believe it happened and thinks about that time and the epitome of how insensitive people can be. (Marian, talking about her husband)

You will always want people to remember your baby who died, especially when you are pregnant again. One father asked his staff to come to the memorial service for their son, wanting them to know that when they were expecting again, a new baby would not negate the life of their deceased son.

> I had the members of my staff come to the memorial service that we had for him. They know we are trying again. (Bob)

How you let people in your workplace know your partner is pregnant again can vary. So, different from your last experience, you may not want to share the pregnancy news with people at work until you are further along. George's staff knew about the loss of their daughter. When they were pregnant again, his wife made a T-shirt that said, "My wife is pregnant again. Be nice to me."

You may find yourself changed in other unexpected ways, too. It can be difficult watching coworkers share news of a pregnancy or birth of a baby. Their blissful ignorance can be tough.

> You never prepare yourself for the second one the way you do the first one. For example, I have a buddy at work. He just got married a year ago, and he just told me his wife is pregnant. And I said, "Oh congratulations. How far along is she?" "Seven weeks." And I thought in the back of my mind, "Oh boy, you do

not know what you are up against." And he was just excited. You could see his eyes beaming. He had already talked to our supervisor about taking paternity leave in July when she's due. He's already thinking about all of that. I don't want to say to him there's a possibility that things could go wrong here. But you think that in the back of your mind. So to me, I look at him and boy he just doesn't have a clue. That just isn't probably part of his world. And that wasn't part of mine until my child died. (George)

If you are lucky, you may have a coworker who will share that he or she has also had a loss. This person will hopefully be further out on their journey and can be a buffer for you in your workplace around baby showers and bringing in pictures of new babies, and they may offer to reach out when you are feeling low and just need someone to talk to.

I did talk to somebody else at work that had just left, and she sent me an email back. I asked them how they coped in their subsequent pregnancy. She just essentially said she put her head down and said we're going to do this. Just got on, and they had twins after that. (Jerry)

Carrying all these emotions can make it hard to concentrate at work. You may have a supervisor who is understanding and will offer you respite from the office space. For instance, when one dad was having a particularly bad day, his boss let him leave to check on property. Other workplaces may be clueless about how you are coping, not understanding that you are grieving your previous baby and worrying about what is going on with your new unborn baby or with your partner in her workplace.

A thought will come into my mind about what happens if she doesn't feel the baby move. What happens if she's at work and I'm at work and she calls me frantic about something? How can we get down to the perinatal center fast enough to where they can save the baby? (Len)

You may find yourself closing your office door and crying alone, never letting others, even your partner, know how difficult the new pregnancy is, keeping your anxiety to yourself.

I do a lot of driving at work, so cry then. I'm usually on my own, so I'm thinking about things, our previous babies, and hoping this one will make it. (Tim)

In your previous pregnancy, work may have been a priority for you, perhaps attending some pregnancy appointments but usually waiting for her to give you reports.

> I remember one pregnancy she went to the emergency room and I had to wait to join her until I finished my inventory. In retrospect, I must have been out of my mind. She had to go through a D&C without me being there. My priority was upside down. Now (in this pregnancy) I try to calm her down, to take one day at a time, to not anticipate bad news until we get it. I think I helped her follow the doctor's advice when that was appropriate. (Jeff)

In this pregnancy you may want to be home more, be more involved with what's going on with your partner and the baby. Increased vigilance in pregnancy after loss is common for most dads. You no longer want to be seen as "just the support person." Now, knowing that babies can die in pregnancy, you may want to attend every prenatal visit.

> That's one thing, you look back and you're like, why didn't I do this or that? Why wasn't I home more? It never crossed our minds, never. I can't let that happen again. I'm not going to let that happen again. I want to be here. (Mick)

If you can't leave work to accompany your partner to the prenatal visits, you may find yourself watching the clock, waiting for the appointment to end to call her for an update.

> Tara goes to the doctor and I call her right up. How are you doing? Oh, he's fine; he looks great; he's growing; he's getting bigger. You heard the same stuff before, so we both are the same way. We won't believe it until he's in our hands, he's in our house. (Doug)

It is not uncommon for fathers to lose interest in work after the death of a baby, and this may be your situation, too. Your priorities have changed, and it can be hard to take an interest in life, even more so in your work. You may not want to work at all or be too depressed to work.

> With the mother there's the bed rest that's required. With the mother you can see the bleeding. With the mother and the baby inside you can see the baby

being physically expelled. I wished I could bleed physically when she had a pregnancy loss, to show people that I'm wounded, too, that I hurt, too. It's like depression. It's a disease, but you can't see it. You can't see the chemical imbalance. It's a lot easier to deal with a back problem. You can't go to the doctor and have him say "I'll take an MRI of your depression and let me put you on some medicine." It's an intangible, a painful intangible that people need to recognize. I was very emotionally neutral, not letting my hopes up until the babies were born, the boys were born. You could never tell. It was a good defense mechanism: shield the pain. (Jeff)

YOU AND YOUR PARTNER

Many women appreciate their partners sharing these emotions with them. This is because she may be misinterpreting your loving protection as uncaring. Sharing that you are emotional as well might even help strengthen your relationship.

> I had no idea that Mike was crying in the car on the way to work in order to protect me from seeing his pain. I happened to hear him telling someone. I told him that I thought he didn't care, and I was really relieved to think that he cared so much, not only about Emma and the new baby but also about trying to protect me. Finding this out immediately changed my negative thoughts about how he was acting. (Jane)

It is more common for fathers to see their partner as their only support rather than reaching outside the relationship to others. You may have learned from your family background or cultural beliefs that you don't share feelings outside the home. This may make it hard for you to express the fears and anxieties you may be carrying.

> I'm not going to lie to you and say it didn't bother me, but I'm not in need of support as much as she is. (George)

MULTIPLE ROLES

You can often feel pulled in several directions by different roles and responsibilities in providing support: a father, and a husband to her. If you have older children, sometimes this distraction is helpful.

The girls are my biggest support. I light up every morning when I see them, every day, every night when I put them to bed. Sure they always test you, they always will, but I get so excited to be around them and that's why I love every minute of it. So that is my support. They're like my rock. My girls make me happy; emotionally, they keep me going. And this new one will keep me going more. (Steve)

Do not be afraid to reach out for more support. Organizations that can assist are Star Legacy Foundation, Sands, and Pillars of Strength.[1] Some organizations have even set up football teams where bereaved dads can meet, play sports, and talk about their experiences with others who understand. If there isn't one in your area, think about setting one up. There are also a few online groups just for fathers. Take advantage of them as a place where other fathers share many of the same experiences.

DIFFERENT PREGNANCY

Your view of pregnancy is no longer a time of blissful happiness. You probably remember your last pregnancy as uplifting and happy but have now experienced the loss of naivete. You mark each week hoping everything will be okay, knowing everything isn't going to be easy and normal like it is for others around you. You are cautious every step of the way. Even when you hear about something new you hadn't thought about before and you are told not to worry, this can cause you to worry anyway. Every doctor appointment you hopefully anticipate good news, and in between visits you worry.

I think it was kind of comparing it to reading a real good book or seeing a movie, and the first time you go to see it you don't get to the end of it. You take this real neat journey through it, but you never get to the end of it; that's the big climax of the story. So then you go back and start the story again. You go through it, and it feels like you're retreading the same ground again. So you're in a hurry to get past all that you've already done before to get to the end of the story. A lot of it feels like we've covered the same ground, and I'm just looking forward to having a baby at home this time. (Mick)

Your needs are also different in this new pregnancy. Your fear that this pregnancy could end the same way because you no longer trust all will be well.

Just like your partner, you are so subjectively involved that you also need as much objective information to know the baby is safe. As often as possible, go to the doctor visits to get this information firsthand.

> Before it was, "Oh, okay, the doctor says this, the doctor says that. It's fine." But now we know, so we're a lot more cautious this time. If something doesn't seem right, she's going in—boom—to the doctor. They're going to do whatever they can to make sure everything's fine. At the same time, we're trying to keep everything as normal as possible without freaking out or being weird about it. The doctors are just more aware of everything now, so we just hope that they can help everything along. We're following this one much, much closer. Even the doctors and Deanna physically pay attention a lot closer to what her body is feeling, to see if anything is different, just to make sure that something doesn't happen again. (Tom)

While you may attend all the appointments in this new pregnancy, you will also need to prepare yourself for unexpected memories of the past. This can happen for you at the first ultrasound visit, where you will be faced with the environment and sounds that you last experienced when you were told your baby had died.

> In subsequent pregnancies there's that association. It wasn't as though we had a positive ultrasound before. All of those same feelings that you have in that ultrasound room—turn off the lights—all of those same emotions, fears, and anxieties, just by the sake of association, they're all you know about being in a room. They all come back, same as going into a hospital and seeing the machine. You can't help but have those emotions come back. (Mike)

SHARING FEELINGS AND STAYING STRONG

It is common that your partner may be your main source of emotional support. At the same time, you may also believe or have been told that you have to stay strong to protect your partner. This can make it hard to share how you are feeling in this new pregnancy. The messages you hear can continue to be "stay strong for the mother." You also may have heard about the research on the mother's stress during pregnancy being harmful for the unborn baby, so you don't want to add more stress.

I don't try to stir the pot. Whether it's good for me or bad for me or inevitable, it's just my own doing. (Bob)

I try to be kind to her, especially after seven o'clock. What can I get you honey? I'll get her water. She doesn't like to move off the sofa. She needs help going to bed. She doesn't like to do the dishes all the time. It's important for her to lie on her side, and quite frequently it's hard for her to do that. So she ends up sleeping on her back at night, and I try to politely remind her to sleep on her side [laughing]. She snores pretty heavily if she's on her back. You know, hugs and stuff. I don't try to bring up any kind of controversial topic. We don't talk about money or anything like that in the evening. (Kyle)

I behave myself. (Tim—meaning he doesn't ask for sex)

Holding back on your own fears and anxieties in order to provide reassurance and stay strong can carry a further burden for both of you. Admitting your fears and worries is challenging and can wear on you.

How can I tell her things are going to be okay? I don't know. It is very nerve-racking, but I don't let her see that. I try not to. I just don't talk about me being worried. Oh, she tries to help. I don't really let her know when I'm worried. (Roger)

Sometimes it can be helpful to focus on the differences between this pregnancy and your last. Doing so helps you recognize this is a different pregnancy and a different baby, a sibling to your deceased baby.

I'm excited about it. It's a little different because last time it was two girls and this time it's a little boy. So that makes it a little different and it's not twins. (Claude)

The second trimester she started feeling better. The similarities between the first and second pregnancy stopped. This is a different path that we're now on. It started lessening the fear of just what had happened before. (Darryl)

REASSURANCE: FETAL MOVEMENTS

One frustration for you may be knowing you have to rely on your partner for reassurance that the baby is still alive. Often this means you will find yourself asking, "Is the baby moving?" This can help settle your fears. It also gives you an awareness that the baby is already here, something you didn't necessarily think about in your previous pregnancy.

> I ask at least once a day. A lot of times now, since I have asked so many times, she'll just say, "She's really kicking away." You know, she might tell me that maybe three, four, or five times a day, so I won't even ask. I don't know if she knows that she's doing that to give me reassurance; I think she just likes to tell me. (Paul)

> What helped me get in touch with the baby was to lie in bed and feel the baby move inside Marci, which scared the crap out of me. This is a living object inside. I don't have to waddle around in funny looking clothes, but this is a living being in there. Each time the baby would move I'd jump—wow. It gave me more of an appreciation for what Marci was doing, her carrying the baby. I don't think I could do it. Every twitch: Is it a good twitch or a bad twitch, a positive sign or a negative sign? Is this the beginning of the end? (Jeff)

The loss of your previous baby has also changed your identity as a father. Even as you rely on the mother for reassurance that all is well, you can also learn to be more aware of the baby, notice changes, and confirm the mother's impression. You can do this by feeling the baby's movement with your hands. Depending on the baby's personality, he may or may not move when you do this. If he doesn't, it can be helpful to place your hand over him and tell him it is you. You can also do what one father did: he waited for the baby's movements after his partner fell asleep. This can be a helpful way to have reassurance as well as a nice quiet time for you to be with the baby.

> I put my hand on her belly and I can feel this one move and kick and kind of roll around in there. I think I'm feeling more attached to this one than I did with Hope just because she could feel Hope move at fourteen weeks, but Hope was never big enough for me to feel the belly move. But I can feel this one physically, he or she is moving around, so I just have more of a connection, I guess, with this one than I did with Hope. (Jon)

You may have regrets that you didn't pay more attention to your previous baby when your partner was pregnant. Your loss has made you realize that your fathering role began as soon as she became pregnant.

I remember Massie didn't move much. I felt her move a couple of times. One
of the times was just two weeks before she died. That's the only real memory I
have of her, kicking my hand that one time. It never crossed our minds, never.
I'm not going to let that happen again. I want to be here. (Roger)

Or you may continue to struggle with being able to visualize that this new
baby will really be born alive. You continue to keep the focus on taking care
of your partner.

I mean, I know I'm a father, but I haven't had many of the experiences of being
a father as the twins never lived outside of her body. I guess I visualize holding
the baby, which I'm not very good at. It hasn't really hit me. I see my wife growing bigger and I know the baby's there, but I am . . . I don't want to say numb,
but my life hasn't changed, other than caring for Ann and what her different
needs are now. (Kyle)

CONTINUING THE BOND WHILE BONDING WITH THE NEW BABY

Now when people ask how many children you have, you may include your
deceased baby, too.

I've still got two kids and a third one on the way. A bloke who hadn't been at
work that long asked me, "How many kids have you got?" "Oh, I've had two."
And he said, "What do you mean you've had two?" I said, "Well, our first son
was stillborn, and our second one lived for twelve weeks and died." And he said,
"Oh, I'm sorry. I didn't know." I said, "No, it's alright. You asked and I told
you." Simple . . . but I still class them as our kids . . . they are sitting on the wall
at home . . . in their little urns. (Tim)

It was really important to me that when my parents talk about their grandchildren that they say they have four, not three, because my brother has three children. I didn't want people to discount her or act like she never existed. When
people ask us if we have children I say, "Yes, we have a daughter, and she was
stillborn. If this baby lives, they will have five grandchildren." (Allyn)

In spite of your continued grief and love for your deceased baby, you want
to give this new baby as much love as you can during the pregnancy. You can
try developing an emotional connection with this baby by doing things that
you will continue to do after he or she is born. You might consciously begin

to engage with your new baby by reading, and through your voice the baby is learning about you as his or her dad.

> We have the storybooks. Read to him a lot. It's kind of hard because I want to feel him move. Stacy was reading somewhere that if I put my hand on her belly, the baby knows it's a different hand, so he'll not move. The way to get him used to that is to have my hand on the belly while I'm talking a lot. We do that a lot, so he gets used to my hand being there and my voice. He'll move right in the middle of the story. (John)

One dad chose a story about the loss of their unborn son's sister, so he would know about his deceased sibling. He felt this was one way he could begin to connect with his new baby while continuing to honor his fathering and love for his deceased daughter.

> We bought a book called *Something Happened* and began to read it around twelve weeks, when we found out we were having a boy.[2] Each night we started reading other books to him. (Naveen)

If you are a music lover, you might try music, as this dad did:

> I rub her belly or I tap her belly, then he'll kick her. I think he does that more because I found certain things that he likes. He likes the guitar a lot—like rock music. (John)

Your partner may also have noticed you are more protective and are now aware pregnancy is a time to be with your baby.

> He's just so interested in learning about the baby. He loves to hear about when I tell him the different milestones that the baby has, and it's just from reading my book. He wants so much to be involved. I never felt like he wasn't involved before, but it's much more of an intense involvement. It's just different. Where before he'd maybe ask about the pregnancy and all he wanted to know is if I was okay. Now he's asking more about the baby. (Deanna)

GENDER ISSUES
Learning the gender of the baby can bring mixed feelings such as disappointment, which may surprise you. You may want a baby of the same gender as

your deceased baby, or you may want a different gender than your deceased baby. Of course, you want a living baby regardless of the gender, but you may feel guilty about having these normal feelings.

> Really disappointed it's a girl. I just had hoped for a brother for Sawyer, who is here. But we make our peace with it. I also think it could be better than having another baby boy after Lincoln. What you want and what you can handle are sometimes two different things. I don't like the idea of a replacement kid because then I have the feeling like someday, when I'm older, I would be able to look back and say, "Well, Luna wouldn't be here if Lincoln wouldn't have died"—really just a nasty way to go about replacing a memory. (Bob)

It is common to need time to process who this baby will be as a separate individual. Learning the gender during the pregnancy gives you time to process your feelings and share them with your partner. This can be especially true if in your mind you saw yourself as the father of only boys or only girls. As this father shares, he was already a father to a baby girl:

> Shortly after losing Sonum I started thinking about what it is going to be like when we start trying again. The odds are fifty-fifty, and I started thinking about what it would be like to not have a daughter with the next pregnancy, and I started thinking about what it would be like to not have a living daughter at all in the future. This was really, really hard for me to envision. While we were expecting Sonum, I started thinking about a lot of father-daughter activities that I'd be excited to do over the next decades. The thought of not doing those things at all was really tough. But something happened when I was in a dark place regarding these thoughts. In a dream, I had a conversation with Sonum where she reassured me that—guess what?—it is possible to raise a girl even if you are blessed with boys biologically: we can adopt a girl if/when we are ready and are in a position to do so. It brought me a sense of relief to have had that conversation with her in my dream. And it allowed me to freely enjoy the moment of finding out, a few weeks later, that we were going to have a boy. Finding out that we are having a boy this time around gave me the same fears that I had when I found out we were having a girl the first time around! In both cases, right after we found out the gender I said to myself, "Oh my God, I don't know how to raise a girl!" and then the next year, "Oh my God, I don't know how to raise a boy!" I'm glad that my conversation happened so that I could

have that same normal reaction with both of my children that most fathers have. (Naveen)

CONSTANT WORRY AND ANXIETY

Your feelings may also swing from "good" to "stress and anxiety," depending on what is going on during the pregnancy. You know that life is uncertain because you remember the traumatic memories of the last pregnancy, such as when you were told your baby had died. So when something seems reminiscent of your loss it can be anxiety producing and you have to get reassurance that everything is going to be okay. Your mind starts thinking about all the possibilities that could happen. You never think it's going to be easy and normal, like a lot of people do with their pregnancies, and are more nervous every step of the way. You may also feel a sense of pragmatism about your anxiety, and you may try to cope by keeping emotionally neutral. This is a self-protective mechanism where you may not want to admit your emotional bonds to this new baby in case he should die, too. There is a struggle between the heart and the head. You may be slow to admit that of course you are bonded to and love this baby, too.

When I think about the baby being born, bringing the baby home, changing diapers, feeding the baby, and getting up at night with the baby, that is still just a dream, or still just a hope yet. So when I think *real*, I think it's more of a protective zone—right now, in the moment, get back to reality. Anything can probably go wrong at any given time. I think I'm trying to protect myself from that. There's no way I can protect myself from that. It's out of my hands, but, still, people will say, "Are you excited for this baby to come?" You say on the outside "Yeah, I am," but I think, in the back of my mind, "Well, we'll see when we get there" because maybe there might be a chance between now and then that this baby might die. (Len)

You can battle with the decision to emotionally attach to your new baby or try to remain emotionally aloof for fear of another loss, as this father found:

It's a matter of, okay, do I fully accept it and embrace it and then something happens, or do I just kind of not get too attached if something happens and it's not as bad. So if you won't accept it or embrace it, it's tough to visualize what's going to happen. Even though you don't know what's going to happen. You're kind of caught between a rock and a hard place. (Jerry)

SUPPORTING ONE ANOTHER

Trying to support your pregnant partner and care for yourself at the same time can be hard. The weight of being supportive can be challenging. You may feel that her needs are more important than yours because you are not the one carrying the baby.

> Most of what I'm saying in managing feelings is managing her feelings as opposed to mine. I'm not the one with the raging hormones, the emotions going up and down, so I'm not the fragile one. I'm not saying that I'm cold hearted or anything, I'm just saying that she's the most important one of us right now. I probably get complacent, things are going good, and then she'll be in a mood and it will get worse and worse. Bad mood for three days in a row, okay there's something going on. I need to be better tuned. (Jerry)

It can be helpful to have a discussion with your partner about what you can do to support her. This may also help you anticipate situations and read cues that might indicate she needs support or protection from someone or something.

> Nobody should know your wife better than you. Watch for cues, watch for the looks, the things that tell you that they just need to be held. That anxiety just doesn't go away for the entire pregnancy. Although there are really strong women, that doesn't mean that there's not stuff. There are nonverbal cues that something's not okay because of the stress level that's on the women after a loss. Pay attention to the stuff that they're not saying. Make sure you're keeping as open a dialogue as possible, talk as much as possible. I could tell when she was having a rough day, and I'd be up cleaning the house to make sure everything was okay when she woke up—the little things that can take a bit of the stress off. And just being there emotionally for whatever she needed. (Joe)

Providing reassurance and taking one day at a time might help you cope, but this can be hard because she's the only one that truly knows what's going on in there. Her attitude becomes your support, so take cues from your partner's behavior. When she worries, it can have a domino effect.

She was like a dipstick in a car. I could tell. I could look at her and know, just by her reactions, she was confident that this was the thing to do, or if there was apprehension. You know when you are on an airplane and there's turbulence? The first thing you do is look at the flight attendants. If they're not nervous and they're serving coffee, you don't have any issues. If they look nervous and strap themselves in, then you have an issue. My wife was my flight attendant. (Tom)

BIRTH DAY

Planning the day for giving birth can mean planning to return to the same hospital where your deceased baby was born. This can be hard because you may not have even driven by that hospital, even avoided driving down the street. All are reminders that you are afraid of what you experienced last time. Therefore, it is extremely helpful to tour the space where this baby will be born.

The actual operating room where the babies were born: I haven't seen those since that happened, so that might bring back some memories when I see those rooms. (John)

It's going to be tough going back to the hospital to deliver, and that's why Tina's got a doula. I'm going to do what I can. I don't know what I'm going to be like. It's going to be tough. It's going to be very difficult. (Mick)

You may disagree with your partner on where to give birth but also understand her reasoning if she wants to go back. This dad describes his reluctance to revisit the hospital where his baby was in the NICU before he died:

I don't want to go back a second time because we were there for a month in that neighborhood, but she wants to go there because it's next to Children's [hospital], so we're just going to go there. (Jerry)

You may be comfortable with the same maternity care provider. This can be especially so if you've been able to attend all the prenatal appointments and thus have had "rehearsals."

I think that was really hard and difficult at first, going back to that hospital where it happened with the girls; just even driving up the same street that goes to it was really hard because it brought a lot of stuff back. I think going there is okay now. We come here once a week, and we're used to it now. (John)

You may also make the decision to give birth at a totally different hospital, regardless of how far away it might be.

The best decision we ever made was going to a different hospital. We drove an hour and a half ride when her bag of waters broke so we wouldn't have to go back to that same hospital. Because what if we ended up in the same room, what if we ended up with the same nurses; all those faces, the smells of the room, everything about that area would just bring that back. That's nothing we wanted to deal with at that point. (Joe)

Just as you may have done during the pregnancy, you will approach the birth of your baby very differently than when your other baby died.

The actual day of the birth can bring a sense of relief for you as well as an ongoing realization that a tragedy may still happen in the future.

Well, it's right up to the moment the baby's born, till the baby's breathing, and the doctor says everything's clear: then breathe a sigh of relief. There's never a rest for the weary, and being a parent, something always could happen. Something you've got to live with— never a point where you'll be able to rest. (Tom)

BRINGING THE BABY HOME

You may be surprised to find that bringing the baby home may be another time for painful reminders and increased anxiety.

Probably one of the worst anxiety attacks I've ever had was bringing him home into our house. I thought, "Oh my God. We have to keep this boy from dying. It's our responsibility to keep this boy from dying—big time." It's really weird, but I can see it. If I ever want to know what it felt like, I look at those pictures and I see myself. And I was scared, scared little man. (Garrett)

While you may have been fine during the pregnancy (or tried to let your partner think you were fine), it may not be until your living baby is home that you become more worried about your baby's health. It might surprise you that you still don't feel secure that all will be well.

Guys are different. It's not real for us until the baby is here. I wasn't bad during pregnancy, I don't think. Once he was born, it got more severe—talk about obsessive behavior. I worried about everything: him getting colds, worried that he was being exposed. It's funny because I look back at that period now and just laugh because it was so obsessive, just over-the-top excessive. Reading was my worst enemy because the more I read the more my brain would start to imagine things. Oh, I'd just dream up stuff, issues he could have. (Mike)

SUMMARY

This chapter has summarized the differences and similarities that you as a father can have from your partner. No one will ever say these are easy pregnancies, but it can be helpful to read that many of the feelings you are having are shared by other fathers, too. You are not alone in trying to figure out how to support the mother, protect your unborn baby, and take care of yourself, too. In the end, do the best you can to rely on each other in getting through pregnancy following your loss. Although you and your partner have endured the same event, your experiences of it will always be different. It is not better or worse, just different.

REFLECTIONS

- How did you feel when your partner was pregnant again?
- What coping strategies do you think might help you during this pregnancy?
- Where do you find the support you need to help with your own emotions?
- Have you thought about the support you might need when your baby is born?

10

The Children

We cannot protect children from knowing death and from mourning by diverting their attention. Protection in this case involves giving them the tools to cope by educating and involving them.[1]

Rarely is one prepared for the loss of a baby during pregnancy. When your baby died, your older child(ren) experienced the loss of not only their baby sibling (if they were aware of your pregnancy) but also the parent they knew before the loss. Your children's behavior is often a reflection of your behavior. They will take their cue from you. It can be hard to be emotionally available when you are grieving the loss of your baby and anxious about the new pregnancy. Trying to support your children in this new pregnancy can therefore be daunting.

In the past, death often occurred in the home, so children were frequently involved. Below is a story from the early twentieth century written to help guide parents in understanding the importance of involving children when families experience the loss of a baby.

In 1916, Sophia Fahs, a Unitarian educator, editor, author, and minister with a special interest in the religious education of children, wrote an article for *Parent Magazine* titled "What Are Our Children's Thoughts about

Death?" She describes a scene in her home after her baby daughter, Gertrude, had died. Her other three children were all under four years of age:

> Before the funeral, a special service was held for the three other children in the family and for those of their child friends who cared to come. In a bassinet draped with white dotted Swiss over which were twined sweet peas, the baby's body lay. Simply and kindly the pastor talked and prayed with the little group of hushed children, and together they sang a child's song.[2]

Before the baby had come into the world, the sisters and brother had shared the joyous knowledge of her expected birth; after she went, they shared with their parents the trust that all was well with the child.

This story illustrates how helpful it can be when children are provided information when a baby dies in your family. Their friends were included with them in the funeral of their baby sister. This gave them freedom to talk about their sister, both to their parents and to their playmates. They were also reassured that their baby sister was safe and that they were safe in their family, too.

SIBLINGS ALIVE AT THE TIME OF LOSS

Involving children in such an intimate way as seen above changed when funeral homes began to take over death rituals. Children were often excluded from ceremonies in a misguided attempt to protect them. At the time of your baby's death, you may not have known how to tell your children what happened, wanting to protect them from the same intense grief feelings you were experiencing. If your loss was earlier in your pregnancy, you might not have even shared that you were pregnant. You may also be part of a culture or family background that has different beliefs in how to honor a deceased baby and ways to involve your children. You may have gotten conflicting advice on how much to tell your older child. Or perhaps your older child was not old enough to fully comprehend what was going on. Yet, in the early childhood literature, it is well documented that very young children sense emotional changes in their parents. You are their center of safety. They may not understand what is happening, but they can sense changes in their worlds, in your behavior, and in the behavior of others around you. Helping your child understand the concept and permanence of death, when your pregnancy ended in loss, is challenging.[3] They were expecting a baby to come home. At the time of your loss you would have done whatever you thought was best for your family, which may or may not have included your older child. Children under three may not have the words for their feelings, but you may have a child who was very intuitive when your baby died. You might have been surprised that your child already sensed something was amiss in your family.

> Grace was three when I had the first miscarriage. She knew about the pregnancy really early, so she had called the baby "Baby Cabbage." We talked about the baby every day. She refers to the baby as her brother, and he is in heaven. The second time I got pregnant, Steve and I did not tell her because the first miscarriage was really hard on her for months and months. We thought, "Let's wait until after twelve weeks, and then tell her." The day I took the test, she just walked up to me that morning and said, "There's another baby in your tummy." Well, then the same thing happened [another miscarriage]. (Marybeth)

Another family, believing they were having a healthy third baby, had an unexpected loss when their son died within twenty-four hours of birth from an undiagnosed hypoplastic heart. In their grief, they did not bring the older children in to meet him. The siblings only knew that their baby brother was not coming home and that their parents were very sad.

> You can always go back and do something better or differently. But I realized in the crisis, you can't beat yourself up at a time like that. I would have brought them down to the hospital but didn't know how to do that. Hank was eighteen months old, so he didn't really have a voice, where his sister was a little bit older [three years old]. She was very sad because we were sad. We did take pictures of Pat and me holding him [baby], but it would have been nice for them to have pictures of him, too, more memories. As they got older, they really liked to look at his pictures and liked to talk about him. They went through a period where they would get his pictures, get to know him, and go through his little clothes that he wore. (Mona)

As you welcome this new baby into your family, children need to be included and reassured that your family is still a safe place to share feelings. If you were unable to share what happened at the time of your loss, either because you felt your child was too young or because you didn't know how, it is never too late. You may find it helpful to share pictures with your children now. This can help them understand what happened and why you might be feeling anxious in your current pregnancy. As one mother said:

> This is just part of our family story. How do you let that be and continue to share in a way that's helpful or healing? (Katie)

PREGNANT AGAIN: WHEN TO TELL YOUR CHILDREN
Just as it can be hard to share your new pregnancy with others, so, too, will you wonder when to tell your children. Telling your children is a personal

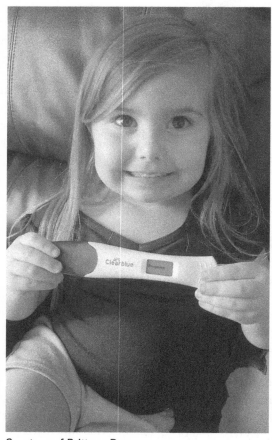

Courtesy of Brittany Day

decision, and only you and your partner know what will work best for your family. If you have a younger child, under two or three, telling your child that there is another baby in your "tummy," when there was a baby there before who didn't come home, might be confusing.

> It's been difficult trying to explain to my two-and-a-half-year-old son that we're pregnant again after previously going through miscarriage and stillbirth. His only experiences with Mommy growing a baby have resulted in the baby dying. I don't think he understands that pregnancy is supposed to result in a living, breathing baby, and he no longer seems as interested in my pregnancy as he did before. (Megan)

When sharing, the information needs to be simple and honest. You have no script, so when sharing information, ensure that it is simple and honest and tailored to your child's developmental age. You may be so afraid of having another loss that you decide not to share until you are further into your pregnancy. However, you may have a child who is very perceptive and already senses you are pregnant.

> She definitely knew [fourteen months]. I remember that she would come and touch my belly a lot. Then when it got closer, she would come and talk to the baby, put her lips right on my tummy and talk to her. (Cheryl)

Your child can have a response similar to yours when they learn about the pregnancy. They also may worry this baby might die. You don't know how the pregnancy will end, so this can be hard for you to hear. Try to give reassurance that you and your maternity care providers are doing all they can to keep this baby safe. It is understandable that your own fear of another loss can cause you to hold back sharing the news.

While you may not want to share, if they already know, be aware that your changed behavior and silence may cause your child anxiety: sensing something is going on in the family and needing reassurance that he is still okay. He may think it is something he did wrong. If your child is between three and four years of age, he or she may be at the magical thinking stage, believing they can change reality into anything they wish.[4] This kind of thinking may also lead the child to think they caused their baby's death by not being "good" or even by wishing the baby wasn't coming at all. For example, not knowing what was going on in her family nor being given information about what was happening around her mother's losses, one adult sibling describes feeling at fault for her mother's sadness:

> I remember when I was three, my mom being in the bathroom. I remember my dad shushing me and telling me to be quiet. I felt invisible and responsible for what had happened. I thought for many years it was my fault my mother was so sad. There was a lot of magical thinking on my part: if I had been better, quieter, kinder, or more considerate. (Meghan)

At the same time, fearing another loss, you don't want to wait too long to share or prepare a child, as this can complicate things when you bring home a living baby.

> I think Jackson had a very hard time when Harry was born because we didn't prepare him for a new sibling because we ourselves were not sure that we would bring home a baby. We would tell him that there was a baby next to my tummy, but we never said anything about the baby coming out! (Christine)

YOUR CHILD'S REACTION TO THE NEWS

Children may not initiate conversations concerning their feelings. Younger children are more likely to show you how they feel through their play, behavior, and sleep patterns. Older children generally have the language to communicate their feelings but may need encouragement to share. Follow their lead in how much information they want and need. Being open and honest is the best way to give reassurance. This can be hard because you also worry about what will happen. Provide information that will help them understand that you and your baby are safe, and they are safe in your family, too. Listen, listen, listen.

> She [four-year-old] was a little anxious about her sister and making sure everything was going to be okay. Nothing real specific. She asked me if we are going to get our baby or if she is going to go to heaven. (Annette)

> We explained to her [four-year-old] that we were going to do everything we can to not let that happen [baby die]. When we go to the doctor now, she says, "You're going so the baby doesn't get sick?" And we say, "Yep, we're trying to

keep it healthy." We say we have good doctors. They're going to do what they can to keep it from happening. (Russ)

If your child is showing oppositional behavior (disequilibrium), keep in mind that it might be normal. It can be helpful to understand that the behavior is not necessarily your child reacting to your anxiety but a normal developmental stage that is challenging and more disruptive. (See ages in chart on page 141.)

Equilibrium versus Disequilibrium

EQUILIBRIUM	DISEQUILIBRIUM
smooth, calm behavior	unsettled, uneven behavior
practicing skills already mastered	learning new skills and abilities
plateau in development	quick time of growth and new development
at peace with self and the world	uneasy with self and the world
more confident	more anxious, more stressed, less confident
a period of stability and consolidated behavior	a period of struggle and breaking down of behavior
easier to live with	more difficult to manage

Courtesy of the Gesell Institute

It felt like she wanted more cuddles and that, but having said that, she was also being a bit more difficult in terms of trying to assert her needs. I think she is probably picking up more of my actual internal stress because she was the one who was being a bit difficult. Maybe sometimes she's picking up more of the changes. Whether she was actually reacting to me or actually being a bit more difficult [because] at three you're sort of trying anyway. (Rita)

WORRYING ABOUT YOUR HEALTH

If you were very sick when your previous baby died, your child may have feared you were going to die, too. Anxiety about this outcome may be more important to them than having a new sibling; look for changed behavior or reactions in his play. Try to ask questions to help clarify feelings he may carry and what your child remembers. Remind him, as awful as those times were, you did survive and are being watched closely in your new pregnancy. If your child is older, you might consider having him attend doctor appointments to see that both you and the baby are being well cared for. Discuss with your partner whether there is a need to consider involving a child therapist if your child is having a particularly hard time. At minimum, if your child is in a school or day care setting, let his teacher be aware your child may need more support.

> Our baby died due to my high blood pressure, and I was also in the intensive care unit after her death. He [four-year-old] asks me every day that I am pregnant, "How's your blood pressure?" I tell him every day that I am being careful and the doctor is watching over me. (Sarah)

YOUR FAMILY NOW

Children usually believe that all families are just like their family. But after you have experienced a loss, your child knows that your family is different from others. It is helpful to have a discussion with your child to talk about how your family has changed because of your loss. One three-year-old came home and told his mother that the neighbor lady went to the hospital to have her baby, "but that doesn't mean a baby will come home." A five-year-old asked her mother why the neighbors were planning a "for-sure baby" when her family said theirs was a "maybe baby." If your child is beyond the preschool years (seven or older), he may understand the concept of death. This means you can expect different and more sophisticated responses around your new pregnancy. For example, seven-year-old Sally's mother's five miscarriages had a profound impact on her, especially the last one that was at sixteen and a half weeks' gestation. From the beginning of the new pregnancy, she was cautious and said, "I didn't really know babies could die until Josie died." During a conversation with the grandparents, her younger brother (five years old) shared that they were having a new baby, and she said, "Well, maybe." She was very matter-of-fact when someone asked her mother what they were having, saying, "We're just going to find out when it's born, and if it dies, we'll find out then."

It can be hard to hear what your child might be feeling, but it is a healthy sign when they are sharing their anxieties. Sometimes your child just needs a hug and reassurance that you are hoping for the best, too. You may also have them hug your belly and tell the unborn baby how much he is loved and wanted in your family.

INVOLVING YOUR CHILDREN WITH THEIR UNBORN SIBLING

Look for opportunities to engage your children with the new unborn baby at your own comfortable level. If you choose to take your child to an ultrasound examination, it can be helpful to bring an older adult along so they can leave the room with your child for you to have more discussion with your provider.

> She's [four-year-old] been up here to a doctor appointment with Sarah. She was so excited last time—got to see her little brother or sister yawn. (Russ)

Taking your child(ren) to an ultrasound may help them engage with the new baby. They see the heartbeat and movements of the baby and begin to understand a baby is really growing inside. This can also encourage them to engage with the unborn sibling with hugs or talking directly to your stomach.

> He's been to all the scans and it's gotten easier for him [eight-year-old]. In the evening, when I'm in the bath, he will come and bring his little chair and sit next to the bath. He'll feel the baby moving. He'll say, "Oh, he likes that story," or, "He likes that bit." So he's very involved. He loves the baby and you know that when you see him. (Julie)

An ultrasound visit can not only help your child "see" the baby but also offer you the opportunity have a discussion about feelings and concerns your child may have. It can be fun to share pictures, found on the internet, of fetal development or affirmations with your children for each day of pregnancy. Your child may also like to engage by feeling the baby moving.

> She's been kicked a couple of times, so she likes to come up and put her hands on my stomach and try to shake my stomach and tell the baby to wake up when it's not moving at that particular point in time. (Grace)

Your unborn baby is learning about your family long before entering the outside world because of the older sibling. Every time you are reading a book or going on an activity, remind your child that the unborn baby is with you, too. Pay attention to how the baby's movements may change around your older child and let him know the baby is "listening."

Sometimes she does this really weird thing. She'll put her head down below, under my belly button, almost around my crotch area, and she just starts babbling up at me. "Are you talking to your brother?" I have Jude's things in my room on a shelf and sometimes she looks up there and she babbles. "What are you looking at? Are you talking to your brother? "If you're here, Jude: hi." It's freaky but it's cool. (Danielle)

CHILDREN'S REACTIONS AROUND BIRTH

Prepare your children for what might happen around birth. If you are going back to the same hospital, consider touring the hospital before birth: helpful for your child as well as you and your partner. You might find it hard going back into the space and have trouble managing feelings that you might not anticipate. We recommend you take the tour before you tour with your child, so you can process your feelings before helping your child. Not processing your feelings first may inadvertently cause your child more distress than necessary.

We thought we would be okay on the children's tour, but it brought back all my feelings of leaving before without our baby. We should have gone first to prepare ourselves, and her. (Dawn)

If you are going to a different hospital, keep in mind that memories of your child being in a similar environment can still bring up many feelings. Remember, children take their cues from you. Remind your child that the people and equipment they will see are there to protect you and the baby. Everyone is waiting for a healthy baby. After the tour, ask questions as to how it went for your child. It is fine to admit the tour was hard for you too.

Also keep in mind who will care for your children when you go to the hospital to have your new baby. If you are having the same people support your child, they should prepare as well and visit the hospital if they can. Even if they are close to the people who cared for them, children may remember what happened around the loss.

Last night was Eliza's first time spending the night at my brother's house since I was in the hospital delivering Sophie and Ruby. When I told her my nieces were having a sleepover, I could see the hesitation in her eyes, and it was different than just being nervous about sleeping over. She said, "Mommy, remember what happened last time I stayed there?" I realized then that she associated Sophie and Ruby's death with spending the night at my brother's house. (Brittany)

Ask whether they want to give you anything to bring along to have in your room during labor, such as a picture they have drawn, or a soft toy or doll. Put thought into who will be caring for your child when you go in to give birth. You will want to choose someone they know, who can understand what they may be going through. Remind them again that everyone hopes to see a healthy baby. When his parents called to say his baby brother was born, eight-year-old Elliot's first words were "Is he alive?"

AFTER THE BIRTH

When your child comes to see the baby for the first time, the baby will know his or her voice and be just as excited to see his or her face as he or she meets the new baby. Your child may be so happy the new baby is alive that they may not be able to let the baby out of his or her sight, a normal reaction for many siblings. Pay attention to your child's reactions because, like you, it may take time for your child to trust that this baby will stay. Your child may also know and worry about SIDS, even if she doesn't fully understand what that is, and may be copying your behavior of frequent checking on the new baby.

You may also be surprised that in seeing a healthy living baby your child may grieve and understand more clearly the loss of your baby who died. Your child may be showing all the signs of being excited and eager to hold the baby but may also be expressing pain and sadness. As your child watches the new baby's development, he or she can be reminded of all that he or she missed in the deceased sibling.

When Tony was about four months old, they started saying things like, "Oh look, Mom. We never got to see Kevin roll over. We never got to see him smile." Of course, it brought the grief back for me, but I realized they understood what they had lost. (Mona)

KEEPING THE MEMORY ALIVE: RAINBOW BABIES

Just as your relationship with your deceased baby does not end, so does the sibling relationship continue. Children alive at the time of loss and those who follow have been described by one research team as "The Memory Keepers."[5]

They play an important role in keeping the memory of your deceased baby, a member of your family, as well as being important in helping the sibling born after to understand the story of the missing sibling. They want people to know they are still a big brother or sister and to say his name.

> My mom had a baby in her tummy, but the baby died. His name was Finn. He's my brother. (Greta, five years old)

Knowing the story about the deceased sibling born before helps children that follow know they are separate individuals and do not need to fill a replacement role.

> My subsequent child is now two and has seen pictures of her big brother. She's asked, "Who's that?" We told her that her brother died and is with the angels. She's been to the cemetery many times. She now talks about her brother on occasion. Out of the blue she'll say, "Ben died, Mommy." Or, "This is Ben's toy." She accepts the idea on her level of understanding, and I like that he's become a part of her idea of our family. (Gretchen)

> Chloe [three-year-old] is very clear that Micah is the baby that came first and we talk about him. I have one of those family necklaces with the silhouetted family with the two parents and three children. (Cheryl)

You may not like the wording "Rainbow Baby." One mother was clear that she found different meaning in the term:

> I changed the meaning for me. My Jude is my sunshine, his passing (storm) is my tears for him; those two combined brought me my rainbow, Arrow. Jude will never be a storm and he will never be something negative or something I have to "weather through." He is my sunshine, me always missing him is my tears, my rain. (Danielle)

As your children mature, they will often talk about their deceased sibling and want others to know about their missing sibling. Your child(ren) may process feelings at school by sharing, in artwork, or when given an assignment about who is in their family.

Madeline, now in first grade, has talked about Bailey, and her teacher said something at our first parent-teacher conference. You know he's a part of our lives and so we talk about him. Baily was her big brother. (Anne)

The teacher approached me: "You've never shared this with me, but your daughter has talked about her brother who died." It was a nice change to share the story after my daughter told her about her brother Flynn. (Katie)

Therefore, it can be very helpful to let your children's teachers know that your family has experienced a loss and there is a new baby soon to be in your household. To find resources for teachers, search your favorite search engine using words like "school," "teachers," "resources," "grief," and "loss." Here are excellent resources available for teachers that you can offer:

Current as of November 2020

- http://www.childhoodbereavement.ie/childhoodbereavement professionals/supporting-schools/schools/#.WnNmf0xFw2z
- https://starlegacyfoundation.org/helping-children-grieve-marian-sokol-phd-mph/
- National Alliance for Grieving Children, www.childrengrieve.org
- Growing through Grief (a school support program that helps children and teens overcome the pain and heartache of losing a loved one)
- National Center for School Crisis and Bereavement, University of Southern California School of Social Work
- https://www.schoolcrisiscenter.org/ (dedicated to helping schools support their students through crisis and loss)
- https://www.dougy.org/grief-resources
- https://www.education.sa.gov.au/parenting-and-child-care/parenting/parenting-sa/parent-easy-guides/grief-and-loss-parent-easy-guide
- https://earlytraumagrief.anu.edu.au/resource-centre/schools-and-trauma
- https://www.goodgrief.org.au/blog/when-bereavement-touches-school

You might also find that entering similar terms into sites like Amazon might give you some helpful resources. Many bereavement care organizations like Star Legacy Foundation, SHARE, and National Alliance for Grieving Children (US), Red Nose Foundation (AU), the Lullaby Trust (UK), and the Irish Childhood Bereavement Network (IE) have helpful resources on their websites. Finally, schools, colleges, and universities might also have useful resources you can search.

Introducing your unborn baby to the story about his missing sibling will be different for everyone, and you will choose when you are ready. You may have already been sharing with your unborn baby why you are so anxious in this new pregnancy. From the beginning of Flynn's life, even during the pregnancy, his parents talked about his big brother, Nolan, every day. Not only did this experience help Flynn's parents separate one baby boy from another, but it was never a question that Flynn was his own little person.

My hope is that Flynn always knows about Nolan and won't remember a time when he didn't know he had a big brother in heaven, so we talk to Flynn every day about Nolan. We may mention him to Flynn here and there, but every single night one of the last things Flynn hears is his older brother's name. When we say nightly prayers with Flynn before bed, we ask God to bless our family and friends who are here on earth and in heaven. We tell big brother Nolan goodnight and that we love him and miss him, right before we tell Flynn we love him and hope he sleeps well. I want Flynn to know that many of our family members are here on earth, but some are not. I want him to know that yes, it's very sad, but it's a part of life and okay to talk about. I hope that always talking about Nolan will make Flynn a more empathetic and caring person as well, especially when it comes to death and grief. Also, I think talking about Nolan so much is also good for us—my husband and me. In a world where people may not want to say Nolan's name, we do, every day, because he is a member of our family, just as much as our living child. He was our first. He made us parents. (Skye)

Throughout your pregnancy you may have worried that your fear and anxiety had a negative effect on your subsequent baby. Always remember, as discussed in previous chapters, your baby was carried in the same space as your deceased baby. At some level, he or she was carried in your grief alongside your loving care. Interviews with adolescents who were children at the time of loss and adult siblings who were born after a loss as well as interviews with parents raising children after loss have found that many of these children have a gift of sensitivity that may surprise you, and it is a gift to the siblings as well as to others beyond your family. When your child born after your loss knows the story, he will ask more questions as he matures and want a deeper understanding of what happened.

> I'm always telling the girls, "Talk to us about it. I don't care what it is, if you want to know more about Sasha." When they get older, if they want to read the autopsy reports, we'll let them. We want them to know everything about Sasha. (Doug)

WHY UNDERSTANDING YOUR CHILD'S DEVELOPMENTAL AGE IS HELPFUL

In growth and development children move through neurological cycles of equilibrium (stability) and disequilibrium (instability) throughout their life-times. To best help yourself in understanding your child's behavior, it can be helpful to recognize typical child development and what developmental cycle your child was/is in, both at the time of your loss and now, in your subsequent pregnancy.

Understanding these periods of growth that affect physical and emotional behaviors can help you gauge your child's behavior. Is the behavior typical of the ups and downs during those periods or exacerbated during the months after your loss and now in your subsequent pregnancy? For example, you may notice your child being more clingy or disruptive. This behavior may

Stages of Equilibrium

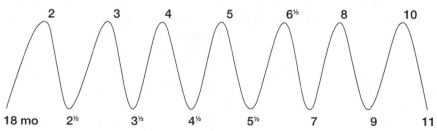

Stages of Disequilibrium
Courtesy of Gesell Institute

be a normal shift in development, which can determine whether your child's behavioral changes are due to your grief and worry. Rely on a family member, a good family friend, or a teacher to help you sort out your child's behavior. Keep in mind that in times of crisis or change, all of us—not just children— revert back to old ways of behavior, to what is familiar, before we are able to regroup to find a new sense of self.

The periods of neurological growth discussed that affect physical and emotional behaviors are seen again, only at a more mature stage throughout a child's lifetime. This means, as your child grows, he or she will be ready for more information on what happened when your baby died. Gesell's theory is known as a maturational-developmental theory. Early in the twentieth century, Dr. Arnold Gesell observed and documented patterns in the way children develop, showing that all children go through similar and predict- able sequences, though each child moves through these sequences at his or her own rate or pace. Most developmental assessments today are based on his original work. There are excellent books written from the Gesell Institute for each year, starting at *Your One-Year-Old* and moving up to *Your Ten-Year- Old*.[6]

Although not researched beyond age eight, Gesell outlined how children may re-cycle through stages and need more information at an older age. After learning about the cycles, one family, whose son died at sixteen weeks gestation, was able to understand how their daughter, then thirteen months (a time of disequilibrium), needed more information on what had happened now that she had reached the age of six. Greta always had a difficult time controlling her emotions, especially when she was in cycles of disequilibrium. Her parents reached out to a therapist, who had not connected that Greta's behavior could be related to the age she was when her brother died. On the sixth anniversary of her brother's death, Katie realized that Greta's body, at age six, carried the emotions of what happened when she was thirteen months old, but her brain needed an explanation.

When his anniversary came around she had a difficult, challenging week. I was lying in bed with her because I didn't have the reserves to deal with the tantrum that night. I was just tearing up and said, "Greta, do you want me to tell you the story again of what happened? Sometimes I think that your body remembers even if your brain doesn't remember or doesn't understand everything that

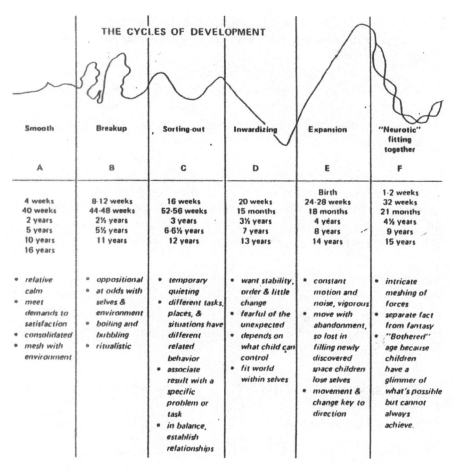

THE CYCLES OF DEVELOPMENT

Smooth	Breakup	Sorting-out	Inwardizing	Expansion	"Neurotic" fitting together
A	B	C	D	E	F
4 weeks	8-12 weeks	16 weeks	20 weeks	Birth	1-2 weeks
40 weeks	44-48 weeks	52-56 weeks	15 months	24-28 weeks	32 weeks
2 years	2½ years	3 years	3½ years	18 months	21 months
5 years	5½ years	6-6½ years	7 years	4 years	4½ years
10 years	11 years	12 years	13 years	8 years	9 years
16 years				14 years	15 years
• relative calm • meet demands to satisfaction • consolidated • mesh with environment	• oppositional • at odds with selves & environment • boiling and bubbling • ritualistic	• temporary quieting • different tasks, places, & situations have different related behavior • associate result with a specific problem or task • in balance, establish relationships	• want stability, order & little change • fearful of the unexpected • depends on what child can control • fit world within selves	• constant motion and noise, vigorous • move with abandonment, so lost in filling newly discovered space children lose selves • movement & change key to direction	• intricate meshing of forces • separate fact from fantasy • "Bothered" age because children have a glimmer of what's possible but cannot always achieve.

Courtesy of Gesell Institute

happened that day." Part of me felt she already knows, and the missing pieces are unsettling for her. I told her about that night. "Honey, you were asleep and my water broke." She had been with me at the ER that day. They sent me home and told me I had a UTI [urinary tract infection]. So she had been with me through the early part, and she had gone to bed. "It was 1:00 a.m. when my water broke. It was really, really, scary. I had to go to the hospital, but we didn't want to wake you up because I was crying so hard. We were trying to be really quiet. We had to leave and wait for Grandma and Grandpa to come to be with you. But I think it was confusing to you. You woke up; we weren't there. When we came home, we just cried and cried and cried. We slept more than usual, we cried more than usual. I couldn't do the things with you that you wanted me to do with you because I was so sad, and my heart was broken."

So I told her the story of what happened: he was born, and how we got to hold him. She asked me a few questions, hugged me, and went right to sleep. The next day, on our way to school, she started telling her sister [Eliza, three years old], almost word for word, the tale, the story that I had told her. It was totally reassuring, and Greta totally settled down for the rest of that week. She knows the story, but now she can understand more details. (Katie)

This example demonstrates how your state of mind and emotions at the time of your loss and in your new pregnancy might give you an understanding of emotions your child may be experiencing at an older age and how your child might need a clearer understanding of the family story.

ALL GROWN UP

Parents can worry about their subsequent children and wonder: Will they be okay as they grow up? You might, therefore, be reassured to know that research has shown that the children born subsequent to a sibling who died, who are now adolescents, typically have three separate views:[7]

1. How they feel about themselves as a subsequent child.
2. How they feel about their parents and they them.
3. How they feel about their deceased sibling.

Children born after a loss often realize they are different. They usually feel loved, wanted, and special. However, they often recall their early years as a time of sadness in the family. They might say that they felt sad or even traumatized when they first realized that they had another sibling, especially if they also realize they might not have been born if their sibling had lived. Interestingly, these children often spoke with maturity beyond their years, and many are working in "helping professions" (social work, psychology, chaplains, nursing).[8]

SUMMARY

Tony's birth didn't change who we were; the grief was still there. It's not like he replaced anybody. It didn't change any of the past. That's a good analogy. He really gave them this huge gift of sibling relationship that they would not have had otherwise. That's really how he lives on and his spirit lives on, the way he's affected their relationship. (Mona)

How you discuss your loss and your subsequent pregnancy with your children, those alive at the time of loss and those that follow, will often depend on your preferences, the age at which loss was experienced, and your comfort level. Be honest with yourself and your children and understand that whatever you decide is okay for you and your family. Comforting and reassuring your older children can be another form of bonding over your lost child and exploring the complex feelings surrounding grief and loss. Your other children look to you for safety and understanding. They may have questions, and you may not have the answers, but you can get through it all together.

REFLECTIONS
- Children take cues from their parents.
- Prepare your child for the birth just as you prepare yourself.
- Your deceased baby will always be an important part of your family, and his siblings will carry the message to others.
- You don't have to be a perfect parent to be a good one. You will make mistakes and can usually go back and fix them.

11

The Couple Relationship

This chapter focuses on the couple relationship, initially in trying to get pregnant, and then in your pregnancy that follows. Just as the meaning of pregnancy has changed for you, your relationship with each other may also have changed. Supporting each other in this new pregnancy can be challenging. You are never the same; yet few people will understand how completely changed you are.

Just as people grieve differently, it is important to recognize you may have different ways of coping. You may cope by using emotion-focused strategies, such as talking things out, or you may cope by using problem-focused strategies, such as needing to know exactly what went wrong in a previous pregnancy or needing to have the results of tests. You may even use a combination of these coping strategies. You may need to see which coping style you and your partner have as they could be different and could affect how you communicate in this new pregnancy. You may even have developed your own code in communicating with each other, as this couple did after their loss and are now doing in their new pregnancy:

Each day is different for both of us, so we try to not pull each other down and still be supportive. Let us be who we are that day. He would message me and say, "It's a rainy day out here," and I would know he was having a tough day. So we kind of had our own way of knowing one of us was having a tough day. (Clare)

As much as possible, communicate your needs to your partner, to know how to help each other. This can be especially challenging if you do not naturally use emotion-focused strategies. You may think that talking about your feelings won't bring your deceased baby back. It may take great effort but ultimately may be worthwhile to improve communication in this pregnancy.

> One thing we've done the best is talk to each other. It's really hard to say, "Here's what I'm feeling." It usually causes the other one to cry. Once we initiated that, we could just talk to each other, be there. (Mike)

As the pregnancy progresses, and may be feeling more positive, you may be the one to help move your partner along. There may be days, too, when your partner is the one who is feeling more hopeful.

> We go slow. Talk about what we're going to do with the baby. Talk about the baby room, talk about putting the crib up, visualize the baby; she starts to accept that, okay, she wants to talk about it. The baby's actually going to be here. Realistically. There were times when she didn't want to talk about it. She'd say, "I can't see it happening." The next week we'd talk about how we want to paint the room. Okay, we've got twenty weeks to go. Okay, then we'd go order something on line. She wanted to feel busy. She wanted to do that so that made her feel better, I think. I don't know. She has a tough time talking about her emotions sometimes; it's tough to get them out. She likes to build up. You can see it coming. You've got to stop her, set her down. Hey, we've got to talk. So. (Jerry)

Being able to communicate with each other is key in moving through this pregnancy. You are aware of the fragility of your relationship around the trauma of your loss and know feelings can go either way.

> It has definitely made our marriage stronger. I'm not going to lie, marriages can only go one or two ways after an event like this, either you end in a divorce or you get stronger. Ours could have gone either way until the night we sat down and had a talk for about four or five hours straight. That night was the huge turning point, the first time we sat down and talked about everything. That was about two or three weeks after the loss. One of the things we hashed out was how I wasn't here. I think we both understood what each of us needed. (Joe)

For one couple, the partner was fearful of creating memories in case their new baby died, too. This may be one reason why partners may resist coming to appointments in this new pregnancy.

> With this pregnancy the two of us didn't bond much together. We kind of kept up that guard, maybe we didn't want to recreate memories of the pregnancy, or something, together. So that part was a little hard. (Kim)

Anxiety is a part of pregnancy after loss for you both. You may be trying to keep your anxiety from your partner. You may think your partner is stronger when in reality they are just as nervous as you. If you can, try talking to one another about how you really feel. You may understand your partner's anxiety, but you yourself are optimistic that this baby will be born alive. This can be helpful in keeping your partner more positive and calm.

> I'm not afraid of losing this baby. I just know. Maybe I'm in denial, but I'm not. He's going to be here. I've always believed that since day one. Sure there's a little bit of me that's concerned we're not going to be holding him, we're not going to be playing. But I see us doing this. I know she's hurt inside. It's very understandable. But I know he's going to be here. (Doug)

You may find your loss has given you new perspective on what really is important in life, and what is not, and brought you closer. This closeness may continue as you cope with the ups and downs of your new pregnancy.

> We're closer now than we ever were before. I think it brought us together, and I don't understand how it affects other people, how they get a divorce afterwards. It doesn't make any sense to me because it was something so tragic that we went through together; it just links you with that person, ties you together for good. If we happen to go our separate ways, we'd be carrying that with us. I don't know how you start a new life with that along with you. (John)

You may have heard statistics about marriages not lasting. Relationships may be challenged and end when couples are unable to resolve their communication difficulties. It is important to realize this can happen for many couples who have not suffered a loss, too. You may never know how your marriage would have gone if your baby had not died.

I remember the night before I was induced [with deceased baby], I just didn't want to go to sleep because I kind of thought this was as much as I was going to know this baby alive. He went to sleep; he couldn't stay up with me. I never could really believe that. The loss actually kept us together longer because I was in a more vulnerable spot. I think that maybe there were problems there that I wasn't looking at quite as closely because we were trying to have a family and that was forefront in my life. Then when we had the twins, I couldn't leave the marriage until they were in kindergarten, and that's when I left. I actually think, for us—just the trauma of everything—we ended up being together longer than we would have been otherwise. He didn't want more children, and that was another issue because I wanted more kids. (Kate)

Understanding your own conflicting feelings of grief and hope in this new pregnancy and then sharing these feelings with your partner can be hard. You may feel confused, and this may cause you to experience difficulty with your relationship if one of you has trouble sharing grief. This can be painful and can feel isolating.

According to my ex-husband, I would stop anybody on the street that would listen about the baby's death. He said that to the psychologist when I went when Jenny was six weeks old [second subsequent baby]. He was very critical of me. And the psychologist said, "Yes, I can imagine. And do you wonder why? You wouldn't let her talk to you. You wouldn't share the grief with her. Where were you for her?" And then he realized what he had said. But he never talked to me about it even then, until five years ago. He said, "I wasn't there for you and should have been. I should have talked with you about the baby." (Melba)

Substance misuse and erratic behaviors may also be used as avoidance-coping mechanisms following unexpected death. This can be particularly true for men.

I remember my father asking me, before I married my husband, if I didn't think he drank too much. I just said, "Everybody drinks at our age," not realizing he was becoming an alcoholic, which became worse after our losses and the birth of our two subsequent children. (Becky)

If your coping and communication styles are creating difficulties for you as a couple, seeking out professional counseling may be helpful. Keep in mind that relationship difficulties and divorce happen in couples who have not experienced a loss, too.

There can be surprises in the depths of feelings that will surface unexpectedly in the new pregnancy. For instance, you may think one of you is not remembering your previous baby when, in fact, there are deep feelings that may surface unexpectedly. If this happens, it can be an opportunity to talk further with each other on how you continue your parenting relationship to your deceased baby while you work together to bring your new baby into the world.

> He didn't say much during [subsequent pregnancy] until the day that Greta [older sibling] touched his [deceased baby] clothes. I think it was with the ashes, and it was the first time I heard him acknowledge to her that she had a sibling. It was funny because for the longest time Finn's little blanket and hat were in this stupid funeral bag that we got when we picked him up. He kept saying he was going to make something pretty to use as a memorial. He wouldn't get it done and it was driving me mad because my perception was "you don't care enough about this to take the time to do this thing." Someone said to me, "This is his healing thing and he gets to do it when he is ready to do it." He did, and he made this beautiful puzzle box that we have some of Finn's mementos in that we got from the hospital. (Katie)

Humor in any marriage helps. In the mist of your fears and anxieties it is important to laugh with each other and at each other about events that can drive one of you crazy. Rob shares a humorous story of his marriage after the death of their first child, born with a severe heart condition:

> I remember people saying that after major surgery or having a sick child, 70–80 percent of people get divorced. I think if you ask Patsy, the only thing that almost ended our marriage was when I decided I wanted to get a dog for Connor [living child]. It was actually a worse thing than having to deal with a sick child. Maybe it wasn't the best dog that I picked out. Patsy's family are not dog people. I could look at it and it would sit down, and Patsy would yell and scream at it and it would just walk the other way or ignore her. The dog almost killed our marriage. In spite of the dog—I can't say for somebody else's marriage—our marriage has been strengthened through the loss of Mitchell. (Rob)

You may also have a partner who uses energy to focus on your older children or projects around the house to keep busy. This is an easy distraction and can be necessary, particularly if you have older children. This situation can be an example of problem-focused coping and what one of you may do to survive the long weeks of this pregnancy.

> We're twenty-two weeks now [time of loss], and that hit Ann pretty hard, I think, but it hasn't gotten through to me I guess. I'm kind of a working artist and I'm making the plaque or memorial for the babies. I'm working on that out in the garage. So I'm still kind of focused on that I guess. (Kyle)

Your other children also may have made you realize the importance of being home more for them and, now, for this new unborn baby. Knowing the love you share with your other children, and feeling like you were too busy with work in your last pregnancy, you may feel a stronger connection to this new baby. You may realize the only time you had to know your deceased baby was at her birth and don't want that for this baby.

> When I found out she was pregnant, I stayed home so much because we knew this would be tough and Tara needs help with the girls. I want to be part of this one more, not be gone. I haven't been gone much this year. Last year I was gone over 90 percent of the time, so I didn't really get the chance to bond with her [deceased baby] like I did with Alex and Sky. And that's why when she came out I really bonded with her within that day. I got to hold her, sit and cry with her. It was good. I felt good. With this baby, it's tough to explain but I feel connected to him. I feel I'm very excited about it. It's just . . . it's different. I'm a lot more . . . I'm connected with him. (Doug)

WHO WE ARE NOW: YOUR COUPLE RELATIONSHIP AFTER THE BIRTH

You will never be the same person or parent that you may have been before your loss. Finding your new sense of self, moving forward with your grief and love for one baby and happiness as you raise your other children takes time. Give yourself time to readjust your couple relationship, and navigate together as you find time for each other now. Of course, part of this navigation is deciding who you feel comfortable leaving the baby with. Sheri shared her story of leaving her baby for the first time to go away with her partner.

> It was just really important that I leave and go overnight with him [Steve]. He kind of moved along faster than I did. The first time I left her [first subsequent

baby], actually, she was nine months old, and I was having a lot of panic attacks. It was kind of one of those things that I think was more for my marriage that I had to go. We had just gone through losing Davis, then being pregnant with Kennedy, dealing with me being stressed, holding her twenty-three hours a day. I had just really neglected Steve because I was just obsessed with this new baby and everything. He needed me to go with him. And it was literally so I could just leave her for twenty-four hours. It was one of those things; once I was gone, I was fine. But then on the way back it was "Get home!" It was hard, but I didn't leave her very often. (Sheri)

SUMMARY

This chapter has focused on how the loss of your baby has changed who you are as a person and your relationship as a couple. Supporting each other through your loss and, now, in this new pregnancy may have given you new insight as to how your life has changed you as a couple.

Be patient with each other as you move forward. Recognize there will be tough periods but many joyful ones, too. One couple has generously shared their feelings five years after the loss of their first child:

We have settled into a life in New Jersey while grieving Madison. Raised two sons while missing Madison. Continued our jobs while wishing Madison were here. Volunteered and tried to help other parents as the only way we know to parent Madison. Never finding out why Madison died has made it incredibly difficult to move forward. Frankly, I miss the man I used to be, and the parent I could have been. Where cleaning solution was simply that and not something that could potentially sicken our boys. Where new car smell was the sign of a well-deserved purchase and not the source of potential cancer [for Sid a new car smell equates to the use of chemicals that may be harmful]. Where each beer was not associated with a twinge of guilt—will I have all my abilities if my kids or wife need me? Where laughing was quite a bit easier. Where the number of kids I wanted to have was not influenced by the number of pregnancies I wanted to avoid. Where baby girls were not a trigger. Soon after we lost Madison, somebody told us, "You will never get over this. Things will never go back to the way they were." However, she also told us we would get through this and come out as different people. That the pain will move from a constant sharp to a shifting dull. She was right. We have two boys, Jackson and Harry, who are the center of our world. Friends and family we are very grateful for. And partners in each other that are strong when the other can't be. But our hearts continue to ache for Madison Yen, who will forever be our beautiful baby girl with a full head of hair and Christine's perfect nose. (Christine and Sid)

REFLECTIONS

- In reflecting on your last months, can you identify ways your relationship may have been strengthened?
- Are you able to list some of the supportive things your partner may have done for you during this pregnancy?
- How have you as a couple dealt with the mixed emotions of continued grief you carry for your deceased baby alongside your excitement of welcoming his new sibling?

Parenting: Moving Forward in Healing

What we have enjoyed once we can never lose.
All that we love deeply becomes a part of us.

—*Helen Keller*[1]

Parenting is always a challenge—more so after experiencing a loss. This chapter covers the many complex feelings you may experience as you move into parenting your baby into his growing years.

> I think the trouble with a loss and difficult subsequent pregnancies might be that those experiences are so hard that parents might make the mistake of thinking that they are the hardest part. Really, we just need to know on the front end that those traumatic experiences and difficult experiences are only the beginning in a whole journey. Obviously, there is so much joy on the parenting journey, too, but I think I made the mistake of thinking Eliza's birth would be the end of the "hard part." (Katie)

Questions you may ask yourself are:

- How long does it take to learn trust that this baby will stay in the world?
- How will your family continue to celebrate your deceased baby while raising your children that follow?

THE EARLY YEARS

Every parent, whether you've suffered the loss of a child or not, can find the early years of raising children challenging. You may find that family and friends continue to be surprised that you are still grieving, not understanding that your subsequent baby(ies) cannot replace your deceased baby in your heart. You always will be parents to all the children you birthed.

> It is normal and healthy to grieve a child you lost. I knew this before, but I especially needed others to know this after the birth of our "rainbow." I still think people expect you to be better, but a new life does not change a life that was lost. I still think about what it would be like to have them both here together every single day. (Melissa)

It will take time to trust that all will be well. Take comfort in knowing all is well for today and follow your child's development in knowing he is healthy. You may feel that you didn't do enough in your pregnancy with your deceased baby, and so you want to do everything possible for this baby. Always remember, your deceased baby understands that you did your best, and you are not a failure.

You may not have wanted baby showers in case something happened. It is normal for bereaved parents not to unwrap clothes or equipment until the baby grows into them or can use them.

> I would only use whatever we could for that moment. We didn't even put the crib together for a while, and I wouldn't let my mom wash any baby clothes until we came home. We washed only what we needed because, even after we were home, we'd go to bed at night and I'd think, in the back of my mind, "He's here now, but who's going to say he's going to be here in the morning." (Diane)

You may feel resentful when others try to give you advice as if you were a "first time" parent and wonder whether other loss moms feel this way too. You didn't get to bring home your other baby, but his life changed the way you will parent forever. Others may think you are holding your baby too much, but it is best to ignore them and do what feels right for you.

> There would be parents who would say, "You shouldn't hold them too much." I never bought into that. I just always thought, "If this is all I have, I'm going to

sit here and hold them." I held them probably twenty-three-and-a-half hours a day, for the most part. (Sheri)

All parents worry when their children become sick. It is understandable that you may be more nervous because of your history. This concern can continue into your child's early years and beyond.

A lot of parents are on high alert when their kids are sick. We were on high alert all the time. (Dawn)

It is important that you find a pediatrician who will be sensitive to your history and understand why you may be more anxious than another parent. When your child does get sick, until you know what is wrong with your baby, it is normal to feel vulnerable to suffering another loss. You need objective data and clear information on what's happening with your baby.

When she was four weeks old, she stopped breathing. She was in the hospital for a week. It was horrid. They were telling us they didn't know if there was anything they could do for her. They were really skirting around it. They thought she had leukemia, which it turns out she didn't. I just remember looking at them and saying, "Is she going to die? You just need to tell me. I've been through this before. Don't give me any crap about stuff." (Sheri)

Even as your child gets older, you may still be triggered back to when your previous baby died. It can be helpful to process those feelings with an understanding friend or professional.

My son was hospitalized for two weeks with hyaline membrane disease, right after his birth, on a ventilator for a week in the NICU, and subsequently did fine.[2] When he was five, he developed a lot of allergies and the doctor said there was nothing really to do about that except get rid of the cat and give him Benadryl. The feelings that I had at that particular moment were similar to the feelings I had when the doctors sent me home when I went into preterm labor and said, "There is nothing else we can do about your pregnancy. You'll just have to miscarry." In both situations I felt like I had to fight for my children against the medical odds. Even though they didn't believe I would have a successful pregnancy, every fiber of my body believed that there was something that could be done. I needed to make an effort and really fight for my children.

I think that's the piece of my parenting that has been so ferocious, fighting still for my children's rights. (Linda)

Although you had much support from your MCP during pregnancy, you remain the consistent provider and your child's first and most important teacher. Advocating for your children never ends, and you will strive to do what is best for you and your family.

If your intuition does not match what the health care provider is telling you about your baby's health, always ask for what information you need for reassurance.

I was labeled a mother driven by anxiety when I was just looking for correct medical information to help my child. I'm looking for them to help guide me, and I don't want to be judged in that process. (Linda)

It is common to worry about the health of your other living children, too. You know how fragile life can be. This may mean it is difficult for you to objectively decide whether you are being overly anxious or if you actually need to go to hospital. Erring on the side of caution and going in for reassurance, saying you are worried because your baby died, will help explain to your medical care providers why you are concerned.

OVERPROTECTIVE OR INTENTIONAL

Does this mean you are overprotective? Protective feelings are common for any first-time parents. Dr. Paul Rosenblatt was one of the first people to address protective parenting behaviors as a normal response after experiencing a loss.[3] Being protective can also depend on your own family of origin. For example, born after a loss himself, one father described his parents as "risk adverse." He was aware this history added to his protectiveness after the loss of his daughter.

The idea of Jackson getting sick because we're on a plane and he's touching everything didn't appeal to me. We didn't take long trips at night. It's okay driving locally but driving further at night was something that didn't appeal to me. We're slowly trying to break that overprotective tendency, but it's still going to be there. (Sid)

The pediatrician knows we are overprotective, but the office has a nurse line, and you can kind of get your questions answered there, a first line of access to somebody to talk to, somebody to alleviate worry or at least say, "That's normal." (Kate)

Overprotective tendencies are not necessarily limited to caring for your child in the first years but are also found in other aspects of parenting: worrying about other children being unkind to your child or your comfort with having your child play with older children.

I freak out more if I think Anthony is in some kind of distress. I worry about him on the bike sometimes, crossing streets where you don't want your kid to cross; you want to grab their hands, fearful of the kid crossing in front of the truck or something. (David)

If we would go to a store, would I let them wander in the store, even in the next aisle? Never! If I didn't see them, would I get a grip of panic? Always! Not to the point where I couldn't function, but absolutely. (Sheri)

My father would always tell me, "If you want to play cricket, don't go on this ground because there are bigger kids who are playing there. The cricket ball is hard. If it hits you in your head, you're going to get injured." (Bal)

In some ways, you will always be more cautious, sharing a common feeling with other bereaved parents. Give yourself time and talk with your partner if you think you may be going overboard. You may understand that being overprotective is probably not helpful for you or your child.

I'm not overprotective. I realized very soon that would not be helpful. Dana was a very spirited kid, full of energy, full of life, had really strong opinions about things, riding a bike, climbing playground equipment. She helped me not be overprotective. (Lydia)

I really know my kids; I'm so watchful of them. So on one hand it's great. On the other hand, I worry that I could drive them crazy. I don't care who you are, everybody's greatest strength is also their greatest weakness. (Fran)

DIFFERENT PARENTING STYLE THAN FRIENDS

Bereaved parents have a new perspective about what is important in life that they bring into their parenting. You are more appreciative for the gift of life, a living child. You may feel a bigger responsibility raising your subsequent children because of your loss. You will treasure your children differently from parents who have never suffered a loss.

> There is no amount of money that someone could have paid me to do anything that could replace what I've been able to do. Even when they're throwing up and get sick and you haven't had any sleep, all I can think about is that they are healthy. This is just a virus, we'll get through it. I feel so lucky for that perspective. (Katie)

> For me there's no choice in the priority. Other people, I feel like they have more choice. That's part of the bargaining I felt I did to get these kids, in that they just always come first. I see neighbors struggling with their kids, but I think the kids are just a miracle. I just want to shake people and say, "Soak it up because one, you're so lucky you have them, and two, it's such a short part of your life that you have them." (Kate)

Priorities about what is important in life as you raise your child also change. Priorities can become simpler, which has worked for one mother. Laura, with a four-year-old and her subsequent baby, now has three requirements for her children as she moves forward:

- Are they alive?
- Are they happy?
- Do they have a life-threatening disease?

You may find others questioning your apprehension or protection of your children. There are parenting and online support groups available with other families who have had a loss. This will help you gauge your behavior and give you ideas on how others cope with trying not to be overprotective. It is also helpful to learn about parenting from a family member you admire who has not experienced a loss and use them as a guide for some of their parenting behavior.

If I had to do it over, I would probably relax a little more, although I did have fun with the kids. (Betty)

LEAVING YOUR CHILD

Leaving your child with others can be hard. Who do you trust? It is not so much how your child will be without you but how YOU will be without your child.

> I remember just trying to go do an errand and just being panic stricken; I couldn't even be focused enough to get something. Part of that was the breast-feeding. I had a lot of fear and anxiety because I had to be there because I had the food. (Kate)

In the early years, if you have an option, you may choose not to go back to work and just be happy to stay home. Even then, it is important to take time for yourself and your partner.

> I stayed home with her, and I probably wouldn't have done that if that wouldn't have happened [son hadn't died]. I went to baby massage classes. I didn't have a babysitter until she was a year old. My husband said, "We have to do some-thing." I didn't trust anybody, so I had a neighbor lady take care of her while we went out for dinner for our anniversary. I was just a doting mom. (Diane)

The challenge is to find a balance in holding tightly and letting others care for your children, too. It might not be until you have more children that your feelings around having others watch your children become easier because they are together and there for each other.

> I think my family thought that my first baby was a momma's girl. I think they understood. But then, by the time I had Max and Isabelle and I was a little bit more willing to let them hold them, they kind of said, in hindsight, "We didn't get to hold Madeline much." So I think that was part of losing one. I was just a little overprotective. (Anne)

Finding a day care provider you feel comfortable with can take time. It is helpful to visit potential places and ask others you know who like the centers their children are at. Some providers may give you a written summary of your child's day. Understandably, you may be cautious in letting your child go on field trips.

> I won't let Elsa go on field trips with the day care. I think that's ridiculous. I may be the only parent, but I think it's stupid: a two-year-old should not get on a bus with strangers and go on a field trip. She's already on a field trip going to day care. (Kate)

It is helpful to find ways to prepare for a babysitter. Ask others who they use and what questions you might ask.

> Within the last two years, with three kids, we have a girl that's right next door. She came over when I was at home and got comfortable with the kids. Now that Isabelle is three and potty-trained, it is a lot easier to not have her do diapers. Usually when we do go out, I still fix the meals, so all she has to do is watch the kids. (Anne)

> Nieces come over when she's asleep, so I don't have to worry about it. I know she'll be fine. I'm more relaxed about it. I just don't want to be gone for days. (Agnes)

MOVING INTO THE COMMUNITY

Transitions, such as moving from one day care setting to a kindergarten or to a school setting, can also be a stressful time. For one thing, you are entering a program that your deceased child should have been in first, so you may have mixed feelings around this event.

Anxious feelings as your child moves out into the world are common. As your child matures, you will learn how to let your child reach out to others and trust all will be well.

> I think my anxiety manifests in different ways now that the girls are getting older. I think it results in a short fuse/temper. I felt so physically responsible for my children's safety in utero and my failure to protect Finn during my pregnancy that it has been hard to let them start going out into the world. They are clearly independent little humans, but I find myself being a much more controlling parent than I would like to be. (Katie)

Check out whether your community has some type of programs for parents of young children: some in elementary school settings, some in churches. Such programs bring your child in contact with other children and you with parents going through similar developmental stages with their children.

> She was really excited to be with other kids her age. I, hopefully, hid my anxiety so she wouldn't see that Mom was nervous. We were just in a room, and there was a two-way mirror, so we were right there if anything happened. And the teacher was wonderful, too. I had told the teacher our history and she was very reassuring. (Anne)

In a group with other parents, you have control over when to share your story. You may be surprised to hear what other parents share.

> I always try to pick and choose who I tell. If there's a mom in there that's pregnant, I hate to freak her out with different stories from my experiences. But if I felt comfortable enough, maybe I shared individually with different moms if we were just playing with those kids and had a moment to talk, then letting them know my history. There's one that has a special needs child. I can't totally relate to that, but I have some understanding. It was nice that she felt comfortable to share. Other ones had miscarriages or different things, so I did get to know them even on a deeper level. It was a safe environment there, too. Same rule that we had with the subsequent pregnancy-after-loss group: you just didn't share outside the group unless it was okay. (Deanna)

Another reason for joining a community program is to monitor the potential of having unrealistic expectations of yourself. Talking about how challenging parenting can be with another parent who understands can be very helpful. It is also always helpful to acknowledge your humanity and allow yourself to feel tired and upset about your baby's behavior from time to time.

Regardless of whether you are in a community program or using a day care setting, communication with the adults taking care of your child is crucial. It is important to follow your child's lead; if they are happy and healthy, enjoying their interactions at school or with friends, they are telling you that life is okay.

> It was hard when she went off to school, but I think we kind of gradually eased into that. I think every year was just a little bit of a growing experience for her

and an opportunity for me to let go. I think we've had good experiences with
the teachers. (Anne)

Each time we tried to change to a different day care it would be a really hard
transition for me. For him it wasn't that bad at all. He was pretty resilient.
(Rosanne)

Build a relationship with the teachers in order to leave your baby. When
you are ready to share, it is helpful for teachers caring for your child to have
your history.

I didn't tell them about my loss until I became close to them, which was months
down the road. They're not going to know that people have gone through
things they can't even comprehend. (Gloria)

Teachers want it to be a good experience for your child. I think if they know
the history, they're fairly sensitive to it. I always told them our history. (Kate)

WATCHING OTHER PARENTS

It can be hard to watch other parents if they have a parenting style that you
envy, or you may want to be the PSA (public service announcement) for parenting behaviors you think are harmful.

I was nursing my baby in a bedroom away from others at a party when another
mom came in with her four-month-old, who had fallen asleep. She placed him
on the edge of the bed AND on his stomach and turned to leave him there. I was
astonished and immediately torn between saying something to this mom, who
I didn't know, and risk being told to "mind my own business," or not saying
something . . . I went with saying something! (Keri)

There are a number of positive parenting courses, books, and resources on
the internet for parenting after a loss that can guide you in setting realistic
boundaries for behavior with your children.

WHEN TO SEEK COUNSELING

If your anxiety around your living child continues and is interfering with your
family life, don't hesitate to seek resources to help. You may be suffering from

postpartum depression and not even realize it. You may need to see your doctor for help in processing what grief is and what depression is.

> Having a living child does not diminish the anguish from losing your other babies. It pains me that for the first three years of Eli's life, I was depressed and, as a result, was not fully there with him. It wasn't until last year that we started to feel like we were moving in the direction of normal, rather than this constant falling farther down a deep dark hole. (Simone)

Never hesitate to get help so you can be present for your children who need your attention now. You may be surprised to learn that sometimes you may get postpartum depression after your second subsequent child is born. This can be because you worked so hard to keep your babies alive during pregnancy that you held back your grief until after they were born and healthy and you had time to process. There are professionals specializing in perinatal mental health issues who can be very understanding and helpful.

> Eight days after my second daughter was born it was my first daughter's three-year anniversary of her birth and death, and I felt I could not express my grief as freely as I had in the past. I suffered from postpartum depression. At first I was resistant to trying to get help. I thought that a postpartum specialist wouldn't understand the complexity of what I was going through. Just as each new life event will change the way you grieve, so too will the type of help you seek. I finally reached out to a postpartum depression specialist; thankfully, she is extremely empathetic, and I have found a medication for depression that finally worked for me, after much trial and error. (Melissa)

> After my third child [second subsequent child] was born—about a year later—was the first time that I actually had time to totally fall apart. I was either blank or crying as I had shut off. I went into the doctor pretty quickly and he was very supportive. Postpartum? She's a year old? But they said it can go up to a couple years after all I had been through. When I look back at that time of raising them, I didn't think I was present. The other day we were watching videotapes of me dancing with the girls. I was very relieved I did that because outwardly they were getting that fun. I had been afraid to watch those tapes or look at pictures because I felt really bad that I wasn't that mom, so I was relieved that I was. (Sheri)

Remember, your children are very resilient and usually forgiving. As you will find in all parenting, you often have a chance to redo parenting behaviors that you may wish you would have done differently.

THE POSITIVES

Of course, all parents love their children; however, the love between you and your subsequent child may often seem somehow enhanced. This may be because you truly value your children from the very bottom of your hearts.

> I have a tremendous sense of gratitude for my kids; I think I cherish my children on a level that I wouldn't have prior to my losses. That's the good side. I appreciate them in a way that I don't think I would have without having to really think about and pray about their lives in utero. The downside is I know that I have worried about them, even just unconsciously, not even being aware of how much I have worried about them, and probably transferred that to my children, even without saying anything, through my attention or my anxiety. Even being aware of it, it's almost that I haven't necessarily been able to change. So that has been the difficulty. (Linda)

> Jackson is so sweet and wonderful, and I assume Owen would've been just as amazing to us. Infant loss creates a never-ending feeling of loss and grief, since there will always be new moments in your life that you wish your child could be here for and the lack of their presence is a void that can never be filled. (Ana)

FINDING TIME FOR PARENTING YOUR DECEASED BABY

Another challenge you may face is finding ways to continue your role as a parent to your deceased baby because for months you have been busy adjusting to your new baby.

> It continues to be such a negotiation of who gets what. Now that Lucian is born I'm worried about giving Tino enough time and energy, so it's a continued negotiation between the two. It's not like I see them in competition, but I just want Tino to have space, even so small. There's hardly anybody that has space in my world right now because he demands a lot of attention, as all babies do. Maybe with time I'll be able to create space for Tino. I hope so. It feels like something that's missing lately. (Karen)

With an older son, I feel like I'm not spending enough time with him, but with a baby who's gone, you also have that layer of honoring them or giving them enough time. If I haven't been out to the cemetery, I feel guilty. If I go too much, I feel guilty. We have a couple pictures of Lily. Some days I light a candle when I feel the need to. (Lauren)

One question that may surface is whether to let your subsequent child wear your deceased baby's clothes. Some parents have given something that belonged to their deceased sibling—things that help honor his continued presence in their family.

We brought Peder home today. We are now a living family of four. We immediately gave Peder his "blankets of love" from his brother Mitchell. Peder is wearing so many of the clothes Mitchell never could. I am happy and sad at the same time. Johanna kept the teddy bear and Peder has been given the good night rabbit and the bear from his brother. (Kathy)

You may also be taken aback by people's responses, as one mother was when she told a friend they were going to share their deceased baby's clothes with the new baby and her friend replied, "Those aren't hand-me-downs. She never wore them." Parents handle this situation in different ways, and it is a topic to discuss with your partner.

John and I decided Ethan should be able to play with his brother's toys because he would have if he hadn't died. (Aundra)

We embroidered his sister's name on some of her outfits for her brother that said she loves him. (Shaylee)

Your new baby will always be a reminder of the sibling who is missing. With acceptance comes the ability to learn to live with this reality in your life.

I think it all started with a book about family he wrote in school when he was ten. He wanted to include Connor but was unsure about how much info to divulge to people outside our family. He also feels very alone because he thinks none of his other friends have lost siblings. We talked about our friends and the histories behind our friendships, of other children who having lost siblings in their families. (Dawn)

Johanna was three when she asked her mother who Mitchell (her brother who died at three months of age) was:

I was surprised that I was able to tell her calmly. She asked me where he lives. She said Mitchell is nice to her when she is sleeping. (Kathy)

MOVING AWAY

What to do if you move to a different home or state and you did not cremate your baby and he or she is buried in the city where he or she died? This is very real, and decisions on what to do can be difficult. It can be helpful if you have other family members who still live in the area where you child is buried. They can be a wonderful resource to visit on birthdays and holidays. Regardless, it is hard to leave your baby behind.

I was very anxious about leaving the house where all our kids had been born, felt like I was leaving Sebastian behind. Sebastian had visited me in the dream to tell me he would be going with us. I picked up the phone. Person on the other end wanted to look at the house. I gave them a time to see the house, called Scott at work, and told him I had just spoken to the people who were going to buy the house, and they did buy it. (Caroline)

You may also want to ask your other children what they might like to bring that is in memory of their deceased sibling.

They picked Matthew's tree because he's buried under a tree in our yard. They call it Matthew's tree. I thought that was cool. (Kate)

CELEBRATING YOUR MISSING CHILDREN

There are many creative ways you may find on the internet to celebrate and honor your continued bond. One is participating in the Wave of Light Pregnancy and Infant Loss Remembrance Day.[4] In time zones all over the world everyone is invited to light a candle on October 15 at 7:00 p.m.

I participate in the Wave of Light every year. It's very special to think that as the sun goes down in each country a wave of candlelight honoring our babies slowly moves across the globe. (Jane)

Another popular resource is buying a remembrance bear. One example is Molly Bear, a weighted bear made by volunteers.[5] They will customize as much as possible with your baby's birth weight and name but may also include other things (e.g., Lauren had her deceased baby's headband put on the bear's head). You can order a Molly Bear from wherever you are in the world.

> They ask you to pick the color and they do their best shot. I love it. The Molly Bear is on Flynn's bed and sometimes he hugs it. (Skye)

Other ideas for remembering your baby include:

> My necklace is an urn necklace. My mom has one and my sister wants one, too. We also have an angel bear with the twins' ashes in it. When I get sad missing Sophie and Ruby, my oldest daughter goes and gets it for me to hug. My mother brought two unicorns. When we travel we take our angel bear and the unicorns—sort of mother guilt of leaving our kids, so it's our way of not leaving our kids. (Brittany)

> I got a tattoo of a butterfly with her name just over my heart. Before I had it, I felt branded by stigma, but now I feel branded by my love for her. (Teresa)

Coping with anniversary times also is something that most parents find persists for the rest of their lives. As you see other children going to school and high school, getting married, having children themselves, expect to be reminded that your child should have been there, too. Further, each family celebration, birthday, or other holidays will remind and hurt. However, it does get easier, as time allows you to gain a different perspective on the meaning and purpose of your baby's short life.

> Bailey's a part of our life and we talk about him a lot. His birthday is on the seventeenth; it's coming up and we usually go to his gravesite and visit him. And the kids talk about Bailey, and we have pictures of Bailey. We have two sets of friends that have babies, one right before Bailey, and one right after, so it's fun to get Christmas cards from them. It was hard at first to hear about their babies. You kind of relive all the sadness for what might have been. (Anne)

> The Christmas following Emma's death we bought a small artificial Christmas tree, and each year since we have added a special bauble or decoration to it in

memory of her. As our children were growing up, they would choose what decoration to buy and then help me decorate the tree. Mike and I now travel a lot and often buy ornaments from different countries to go on the tree. There are ornaments from the United States and Europe, even the Arctic! Last year one of my granddaughters was old enough to help me put all the decorations on the tree, such a lovely special moment. (Jane)

If your deceased baby/child had special needs, many people will mistakenly think, at some level, that you are relieved that the baby is at peace. However, whatever the circumstances around your baby's death, you are never done with grieving the loss of your child.[6] Five years after the loss of Mitchell and watching her two healthy children's development, this mother has a better understanding of how sick her son was when he died:

I thought that in April of this year I was doing very well, but summer and fall have been difficult for me. Each day and date match just as if it were five years ago. I can think of every detail in Mitchell's life. Two years ago, I watched Mitchell's videotape and I grieved because I never really realized how sick he was. His human body had many deformities. I never saw them before. I cannot believe it took me five years to see that. I have decided this will never be "over," at least while I am on this earth. I will always be learning from Mitchell's life. I feel like people are now thinking "Get over it and move on," so I search for anyone who will talk to me. I will always have moments of profound grief and I need to allow myself to have that. There is no reason to stop or try to change it. (Kathy)

Years out you may have your own private memories of finding meaning that you may choose only to share on a social media site or with your subsequent child.

My arms still hold that heaviness and emptiness of leaving the hospital without my daughter, twenty years later. (Polly)

My daughter Sarah, who was born one year after her big sister Emma's stillbirth, is now twenty-five and a social worker. Recently, a high-profile couple had a "rainbow" baby, and they gave her the same middle name as their baby who had died. I was away at the time, but our text conversation went like this:
Sarah: What do you think about her middle name?

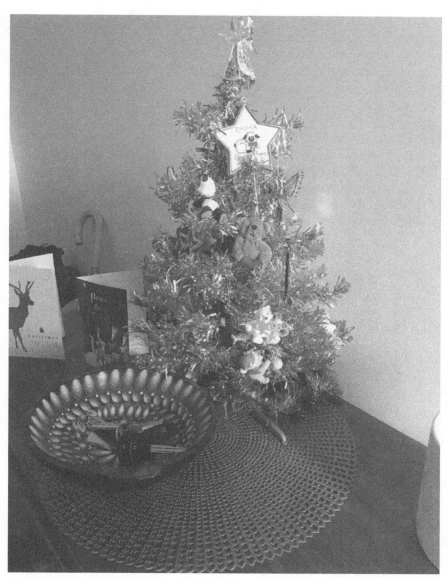

Courtesy of Jane Warland

Me: Pretty common.

Sarah: For rainbow babies?

Me: Yes, but how would you feel if your middle name was Emma?

Sarah: I think it would be a constant reminder of what we lost [note use of "we"]. Not sure if it would be a burden or a legacy; I guess it depends on the parents' mindset. (Jane)

Fast forward nearly nineteen years, and the memory has been transformed into something more like gratefulness. I post his age every year on his birthday on Facebook, and those who know just give it a heart. It's ENOUGH. I keep a plant alive—and I have no green thumb. But I'm comfortable saying I have FOUR children and saying a secret "sorry" to him in Heaven. He was never mine. He always belonged to God. (Suzanne)

SUMMARY

Kathy Haugen shares what she did differently as a parent with her two subsequent children after her son Mitchell's short life.[7] You may find these suggestions helpful:

1. We put a single bed in the kids' room so that I could go in there and be near them during the night if I needed to, without disturbing them. It was such a comfort to me.

2. I would go into their rooms when they were babies, and I still do, to kiss them or touch them. I never worry about waking them up or messing up their sleeping schedules. It always seemed like when I needed to touch them, they must have needed me, too, because they would fall into a deeper sleep. I think if Mitchell wouldn't have died, I would have been stricter with myself, thinking that they needed a schedule. To tell the truth, we have the best-sleeping kids to this day!

3. We talked about when I tell people I have three kids or two. The other thing I did was put all three baby rings on a necklace. I wear that necklace almost every day. For me that is how I am okay with saying that I have two children, because I know that I am "wearing" my three children over my heart.

4. Johanna never knew how I struggled with that question, and one day she told me that Mitchell had talked to her in her sleep and told her that she is the oldest and that she could say she was the oldest in the family.

Ripple Effect:
Families and Friends

The loss of your baby can have a ripple effect on other people in your life: your adult siblings, parents, grandparents, and friends. Dealing with your family and friends may feel difficult at times. This effect continues when you enter a new pregnancy. Taking on the work you need to do in coping with your own fears and anxieties in this new pregnancy while others are just wishing you would be happy again is confusing. They simply don't understand what it is like, and you must not expect that they can. In this chapter you will hear both positive and negative messages, as well as helpful ways to respond and how to get your needs met.

THEY DON'T UNDERSTAND

People, in general, are uncomfortable around others who are greiving. Our society is not good at giving people the time needed to grieve, even more so when you're grieving the loss of a baby, who some may even say you didn't know at all. While some of your family and friends will understand how drastically the loss of a baby has changed who you are, others will not. This can be exhausting.

Comments from others may surprise you, even when you share that you are trying again or if you're pregnant again. If you already have healthy, living children, many will believe you should be happy with what you have now and not try again.

It was difficult because a lot of people didn't basically expect us to get pregnant again. (Rachael)

Some people believe that once you achieve pregnancy you will "finally" stop grieving and be your old self again. Family and friends want you to move on and just be happy that you are pregnant again. They usually don't understand that you wish you could be carefree too.

Because people go, "Oh my gosh. I'm so excited for you. That's so great." I'm like, "Okay, you can turn it off now. You don't have to overcompensate. You're freaking me out." It's just always interesting who says something and who doesn't, who's there for you and who's not. (Allison)

Unless you are around others who have suffered a loss, it can be hard for some to understand that this new pregnancy does not take away your grief. Indeed, it is a constant reminder of your pregnancy with your previous baby and can add a new layer of sadness. You may tire of hearing "everything will be okay this time." But they don't know that everything will be okay, and neither do you. You carry confusing feelings in wanting another baby while missing your deceased baby, what one mother called "excess baggage."

Bear in mind that family and friends generally don't understand. There is, overall, a general lack of understanding of what parents endure during their next pregnancy. You may also be frustrated by people who think your new pregnancy will fix everything. They may wonder how you can feel anxious when it was your choice to try again.

The only advice you can offer to family and friends is to just listen and be there. You don't want to hear that everything will be all right because it may not be. This can make you feel isolated and misunderstood. We suggest that family and friends be asked not to say "everything will be all right this time" because no one can know that for sure. Better that they be asked to appreciate that you will not feel reassured until your baby is born alive. It is also not helpful for your family and friends to tell you to be "more positive" about the pregnancy, as this isn't usually possible after your previous experience of pregnancy loss.

FINDING SUPPORT

Getting support from others may be very different from your last pregnancy. Before your loss people were excited for you, wanting to be kept updated, and may have planned a shower for you. After your baby died you may have been surprised at the number of people you thought were "friends" who were unable to deal with your loss and now don't know what to say.

> The first pregnancy, they [friends and family] wanted to be there for you and go through it with you. This time, if you want the support, you have to call and bring up the conversation with them. (James)

> We seemed to get a lot more calls the last time, support from a lot of people: "Congratulations. Keep us updated on it." A lot of people were excited about it. This time we don't hear a lot about it from distant friends. We still hear from family that is real close, but the other ones are kind of distant. I don't think they're being mean about it or anything; I just think they don't know how we'd take it. So they're just careful what they say, or they don't say anything. They just avoid it all together. (Doug)

> I find that some of my family members don't want to bring it up because they don't want to hurt my feelings. They don't want to make me cry. But yet I need someone, you know, to listen to me. I think that's the only way you heal is by talking about it. So that's been frustrating. I find if I bring it up and talk about it that they're more apt to talk about it a little bit more. (Rochelle)

WHAT ABOUT THE GRANDPARENTS?

A pregnancy that follows loss can be an emotional experience for other family members, too. They also will have many feelings when hearing you are pregnant again. Family members understand that having another baby can be a blessing, but this does not take away the past. They will have their own feelings and reactions in this new pregnancy. When your baby died, they not only grieved the loss of a grandchild but also felt helpless while watching you grieve. You may remember the faces of your parents or siblings when your baby died, and you may have felt some responsibility for their grief. It can be hard for you to deal with their reactions when you are having your own fears and anxieties.

Keep in mind that your parents (the grandparents) have often been described as forgotten mourners. Even their friends want them to "stop talking about their deceased grandchild."

> I feel alienated because there's no one else to talk to. I don't know if you've noticed, too, that friends you had before this child was born, if they had a grandchild that was born even a year either direction of this, after a while the friendships kind of slip away, and they're thinking, "They're still talking about that baby?" (Grace)

They need support but don't want to burden you.

> As a grandparent there is a deep and profound feeling of helplessness. You can't make it better and you can't take your child's pain away. All you can do is witness and hope your child opens up to you. (Lynn)

> You're hurting so bad yourself, but you hurt for your parents, too, because they lost a grandchild. You feel like sometimes you're putting your grief aside to help them deal with it. And you feel like you shouldn't have to do this. So sometimes it's so confusing. (Rochelle)

You may have parents who experienced the loss of children themselves. This sometimes can help as they can identify with your feelings. Be aware that their own grief will resurface, making it harder to get support in the beginning. Or you will have parents who confirm that, even with a new baby, you will always have your deceased baby in your heart.

> When my mom and dad found out about it, it was like, for my mom, all the memories just came back to her and my dad. And that's why it was very tough for them. (Doug)

You may also have a grandparent who doesn't understand or is confused as to why you are not embracing this new pregnancy and baby. It can be hard for them to understand that this growing baby is a constant reminder of your loss and the love you had for your previous baby.

> I worry that she is not excited about this new baby. She doesn't want to talk about it to me and doesn't want me to bring it up. (Betty)

You may initially think family members are being insensitive, but be aware there may be underlying feelings that they don't understand themselves. Grandparents worry about another loss and what this might do to you. They want to protect you from ever hurting again, but can't, and do not want to see you go through the pain of another loss.

> My dad: basically old style, basically typical male, happy, very happy. My mom, on the other hand, she's an emotional basket case. You mention anything about it, she's bawling. She cries because she's happy that it is going well. They don't want to see us go through it again. But it's still there—the support. (Russ)

> I'm pregnant again and my mother will not let me share the news with my three- and four-year-old. I think it's because it is too scary for her. (Joy)

You can experience a range of feelings from your parents. Your parents may not know what to say when you announce this new pregnancy. They want to be happy for you but also worry that if they say the wrong thing, it will upset you. The grandparents may worry about your health, medically, as the mother, if your last pregnancy was high risk, as well as your emotional needs as a couple. It can be hard for your parents to be on the sideline and not be able to share all their fears, too.

> My daughter's last pregnancy was a stillbirth at six months' gestation. Her blood pressure dropped and there was a fear that we might lose her, too. I felt very helpless and profoundly sad. Even though she has now had one successful pregnancy, I must admit that the thought of her going through another pregnancy fills me with fear, not only of another baby loss but of losing her as well. (Lynn)

You may not find their comments helpful. You may sense anger that you are even trying again. They don't want to see you go through another loss or may have difficulty dealing with their own fears or grief. All you can do is reassure them that you and your health care provider are managing your pregnancy.

> Well, my mother's been like a worrywart for me, too. That's been interesting. I said, "My doctor said to cut down the activities." Her response was, "Well, you better cut everything off your social schedule until this baby is born." Okay,

Mom. I'm glad you don't live in the same town because you'd come over here and make sure I stayed under house arrest, basically. So my mom's been overly protective. Fine, that's a mother. I can understand that. (Allison)

She's all excited about it. She wants to know every day how I'm feeling. She said, of course she wanted the baby to be fine, but her greatest concern was me. So yes, she's really excited about this. We both regret that we don't live closer together. (Kelli)

It is important to talk with each other about how you will handle comments that aren't helpful and embrace the ones that are. Decide as a couple how you may want to deal with others' feelings and comments in this pregnancy.

My family was just overjoyed, so happy for us. My mom got tears of joy in her eyes. My husband and my mother have been the two greatest supports in this pregnancy. (Rochelle)

As with our other two losses we quickly pick ourselves up and try to move on. Well, it seems like, especially after this baby, some people (especially my mom) have little understanding for this reaction. I have heard the words "being selfish" thrown at me for putting myself "at risk" and bringing people down with me/us in case this happens again. I understand that a lot of these feelings are my parents being worried about me, but there has to be a better way than making Colin and I feel guilty. (Vicki)

Unlike your previous pregnancy, you may hesitate to share information in this new pregnancy. You don't need their worry as well, and so you so may protect your parents or in-laws from too much information. This is common.

If you were to share with the family everything that's going on in the pregnancy, next thing you'd hear, "Oh, you should get another doctor. You should get a second opinion. You shouldn't listen to that doctor. You can't listen to all that." So we kind of watch what we say around family and friends in this pregnancy—not that we're hiding it. We have to stay focused on this pregnancy, and to hear all these unsolicited remarks just gets your anxiety level up. So this time around, with this pregnancy, I've just learned to ignore family and friends, what their opinions are: it's a girl if you're carrying it high; it's a boy if you're carrying it low, all that crap. I don't listen to that anymore. Every two weeks I listen to what the doctors have to say at the perinatal clinic and go from there. (Len)

We'd love to share everything, but you just kinda know it would be better for both of you if you don't give them quite the whole story. You know, not that we lie or hide anything from them. But there's just, you know, details they are probably better off not knowing. (Sarah)

Grandparents can also worry about raising your new baby in the shadow of your deceased baby. If you are lucky, you will have parents who can play an important role in keeping the memory of your deceased baby alive while celebrating the new sibling as a unique person in his or her own right. It is important that family members, such as your adult siblings, understand what you have gone through and can help support their children, the cousins, in remembering your deceased baby, too. One set of grandparents bought the book *Something Happened* for their other grandchildren to help that family understand what happened to their aunt and uncle and to know about their deceased cousin.[1] When the subsequent child was born, one three-year-old cousin said, "Oh Grandma, now I get to hold this baby, but my baby cousin is always in my heart."

You may be pleasantly surprised at how some cousins can be protective of your deceased baby.

When my oldest sister's three boys found out I was pregnant, they were very concerned about where this new baby was going to sleep, pushing in on Derik's territory and its relationship with Derik. They said, "Where's the new baby going to sleep?" I said, in the nursery, in the baby room, across from my room. And they said, "Derik's room?" And I said, "Well, I think Derik would be willing to share the room, don't you?" And they said, "Yeah." It was kind of neat coming from their little perspectives, of six, ten, and twelve. (Susan)

CHANGED RELATIONSHIPS

Taking care of yourself and keeping relationships that were once important to you often changes after your loss. This is painful but not uncommon. You may have had to deal with grandparents or friends who won't talk about your deceased baby, hoping you will just move on with a new baby.

When we were on a trip in May it was my son's birthday. This is also the day that his first daughter was born dead in 2015. Even though they have a beautiful subsequent baby, I guess I wanted to feel that it was all okay now and perhaps they were not still hurting. I know better. I know that the child who isn't there never really leaves your mind, but I didn't know how to bring it up. It seems to me that it is important for parents and their children to dialogue on how they would want us to talk about it. (Lynn)

You may regain friendships after your baby is born. Or you may never again feel close to a person to whom you were previously attached. One grandmother shares the difficulty she has experienced in watching her two daughters-in-law who were so close before the loss:

When my son's baby died, my other son's wife was also expecting a baby at the same time, about six weeks from delivery. It was very painful for her to be at the cemetery when Anna died, and she was carrying a healthy baby and was not having any problems. After the baby was born, Dana would not come around and would not attempt to see him because I'm sure it was very painful for her. Then Dana became pregnant after Anna, within three months, so the cousin was about two months old when she became pregnant. It created a real tension. Sarah felt almost guilty that she was able to have this healthy baby, knowing that Dana had lost Anna. So she grieved that, but I think she also grieved because she didn't have the relationship with Dana anymore. (Sheryl)

You can help your parents and adult siblings find ways to be more supportive by encouraging them to join an online support group just for grandparents and extended family members.[2] In such a group they will connect with other family members who also have adult bereaved children/siblings. They learn from each other how to cope, what to say, and what is not helpful for you, both at the time of loss and in your new pregnancy. They are aware of how often they say the wrong thing and learn from each other what worked and what didn't. This is especially helpful not only for you but also for them if your parents or siblings live a distance from you.

WITHDRAWING TO PROTECT YOUR EMOTIONS

Although pregnant with a new baby, another effect that may surprise family and friends is protecting yourself from events or activities. Another common theme you may struggle with is what to do with your adult siblings (or close friends) who are also pregnant or just had their own baby. Grandparents may have to find balance in supporting you but also wanting to be happy and joyful for a grandchild already here, one whom you might not want to even see until your own baby is born alive. You have control over how long you might wait to see a new niece or nephew; one mother reported her nephew is eight months old and she still has not seen him. You may also have an adult sibling who feels guilty that he has his healthy baby and you do not.

While you may find much support from family and friends, you may also be surprised and caught off guard when someone is insensitive to your situation. This can be especially difficult around holidays, baby showers, or any event where you might see babies or pregnant women. To some people it may appear that you are making "mountains out of molehills." They want you to be okay and happy again, not understanding that grief for your deceased baby is part of the journey. It does not go away just because you are pregnant with a new baby. Most painful can be encountering people, especially family members, who discount the meaning of your loss by not acknowledging that you are already parents.

At Easter we were pregnant already, but nobody knew. One of his sisters made a comment: "When are you going to start having babies?" I don't know what she was thinking. It felt very insensitive. We actually delivered a baby. It hurt when people would say, "Oh, you had a miscarriage" because it wasn't a miscarriage to me. No, I had this baby, I held her. That one comment, I don't know if it was a slip or what, but I reacted, I told her, "We have tried." Everybody else in the room, their mouths dropped. My husband wasn't in the room when that comment came, and I think she realized she said something wrong. Everybody switched topics at that time. But a couple of his sisters have been supportive, ones we're a little closer to. (Deanna)

With this one we're not thinking about family vacations. My brother's getting married in October, so my parents are all telling people, "Oh, Stacy's going to have the baby at the wedding." There was no future with the girls, so to think there might be one with this one is hard. It's weird. (John)

We've done a very good job of isolating ourselves from anybody with children. For our friends that have children, we don't see them. Any babies that were born at the time that Nicolas was born, or after, we don't see them. So the point of all that is, I'm afraid that because I've isolated myself and I've put up those barriers for so long now, all of those emotions that I've been failing to deal with, that I've been suppressing, are really going to hit me when the baby comes. (Debbie)

Keeping your deceased baby as an important part of your family may be crucial to you. That said, some people around you may not understand your wish to display and share your memorabilia. Or you may have parents (grandparents) who never forget your deceased baby is an important member of the family. You may be grateful when your baby is included as you are pregnant with his or her sibling.

It was really important to me when my parents talk about their grandchildren that they said they had four, not three, because my brother has three children. I didn't want people to discount her or act like she never existed. I did not want that, and my parents have been great about that, keeping her memory alive. When people ask us if we have children: yes, we have a daughter, and she was stillborn. (Deanna)

You may have relatives who understand you are still parents to your deceased baby, who remains an important member of your family.

The necklace was a gift from my parents. When my mom was here with us after the birth, she called my dad and asked him to get a necklace made for me. He went to the jeweler and worked with them to design my necklace, and also an angel to add to my mother's "grandmother" necklace. He tells me that it was one of the hardest things he ever had to do. The necklace is extremely special to me for many reasons, but knowing what my dad put himself through to do this for me makes it even more special. (Deanna)

My mom thinks of me already as a parent. You know the cards like "parents-to-be"? We will be called parents-to-be instead of parents. Even if this was our first baby, we'd be parents. But we already are parents. We already have a baby. (Janelle)

ADULT SIBLINGS

You may be fortunate to have siblings who understand how difficult this pregnancy may be for you and who check in frequently.

> My brother said to me early on in the pregnancy, "I'm not going to ask you every day because that gets annoying, so you tell me what's going on." He and I talk a lot during the week, but he has made a couple extra phone calls just to check to make sure I was doing okay. In part because he knows if my mom can't get ahold of me, she's going to call him next [laughing] and find out what's going on with me. (Stephen)

> My sisters have been really great. I know they're always there if I want to call and talk to them. They wait for you to make the move and take their clues from me. They'll ask, "How's everything going?" You know, you can tell they're talking about the pregnancy, and I'll just say everything's fine and go on to something else. (John)

You may know only too well that loss can change many things within your own family. Even if you have adult siblings who have never been pregnant, they also know babies can die. You may have adult siblings who fear having their own children because of your losses. It is important to not take on other people's fears and anxieties and have heathy boundaries for yourself.

> My sister never had babies, and I think watching the experiences that I went through influenced the process. They tried to get pregnant for years. She had gotten pregnant one time and she miscarried at thirteen weeks. Then she decided to adopt. (Kate)

> For me it's hard because I'm at the age where I want to start a family, and I'm worried about it. It's been hard to talk to her [sister] about it because I was trying to get pregnant while she was pregnant with her baby that died. We don't really know what the condition is [that caused the losses]. (Joy, adult sibling)

If you have older children, you may be surprised to hear them say they will never have children when they grow up. They have lost their innocence around pregnancy, too.

My sixteen-year-old son said he is never going to have children. His eleven-year-old sister agrees. (Tanya)

Even though you are pregnant again, hearing news that another family member is having a baby can be hard. It is important that you discuss with your partner how to navigate your feelings.

He's [husband] talking to her [husband's sister] on the phone, and he's mouthing to me, "She's calling to say she's pregnant." I said, "I don't want to talk to her," and I got on my bike and rode to the cemetery, which was five miles away, and I cried the whole time. And cars stopped. "What's the matter?" "Just leave me alone." So, I biked ten miles that day to the cemetery and back just because my sister-in-law called to say she was pregnant. I couldn't believe it. (Diane)

I have a sister who I've never had a very close relationship with. Once Nicolas passed away she decided she wanted to have a baby, and she did, immediately. So nine months after I buried him, she had hers. When she knew she was pregnant, before she told me, she asked me if it would be okay if she had a son someday and named it Nicolas. Even though I'm pregnant again, I'll never forget that, or the way that she behaved toward me when I was upset. And she said, "The world doesn't revolve around you. Am I supposed to put my plans on hold for you?" (Debbie)

My brother is not helpful at all, not at the time our son died or now, in our new pregnancy. He didn't even call me. He never called me for over two months. He finally sent me a letter. (Steve)

Holding a new nephew, niece, or friend's baby can also be difficult. You have the right to decide whether you are ready to do that.

Allyn was fine with it. He held the baby right away. I, of course, couldn't. They asked. They understood, but I just couldn't, I just couldn't. Even at that point, I was pregnant, but it was just too early. It was hard, but it's become easier. (Deanna)

My husband's brother and his sister-in-law conceived their third child right after we conceived Nicolas. They had a healthy baby, and when we lost our baby, it freaked them out too much to call us. They couldn't handle it, so they never did. And to this day, my sister-in-law has yet to contact me. And how great is it that she sends me pictures of the kids at Christmas? I don't want to know how big her baby is. I don't want to see her even though I'm pregnant again. It's really hard. (Debbie)

SUMMARY

Navigating a new pregnancy with those around you can be a challenge. It is important that you protect yourself from those who do not understand what you are going through and embrace those who are supportive and helpful. You may even find it helpful to express your feelings with those who try to say the right thing but can't seem to find the right words. It's okay to acknowledge to those who love you that sometimes just holding your hand or giving you a hug is enough.

Notes

CHAPTER 1

1. M. Leunig, *The Prayer Tree* (New York: HarperCollins, 1998).

2. Michael Trout, Infant Parent Institute, Champaign, IL. MTrout@infant-parent.com.

3. Susan Schuster Campbell, *Called to Heal: African Shamanic Healers* (Twin Lakes, WI: Lotus Press, 1989).

CHAPTER 2

1. https://www.goodreads.com/author/quotes/6466154.Kahlil_Gibran.

2. Annette K. Regan et al., "Association between Interpregnancy Interval and Adverse Birth Outcomes in Women with a Previous Stillbirth: An International Cohort Study," *The Lancet* 393, no. 10180 (2019): 1527–35.

3. L. B. Shettles and D. M. Rorvik, *How to Choose the Sex of Your Baby: Fully Revised and Updated* (New York: Harmony Books, 2006).

4. "Natural Ways to Boost Fertility," accessed June 16, 2019, https://www.medicalnewstoday.com/articles/324411.php.

5. T. Attig, "Relearning the World: Making and Finding Meanings," in *Meaning Reconstruction and the Experience of Loss*, edited by R. Neimeyer (Washington,

DC: American Psychological Association, 2001), 52. See also https://www.
lifeanddeathmatters.ca/thomas-attig-the-heart-of-grief/.

CHAPTER 3

1. J. O'Leary, "Grief and Its Impact on Prenatal Attachment in the Subsequent
Pregnancy," *Archives of Women's Mental Health* 7, no. 1 (2004): 1–15.

2. https://starlegacyfoundation.org; https://pregnancyafterlosssupport.org.

3. The antiphospholipid syndrome is a disorder of the immune system that
is characterized by excessive clotting of blood and/or certain complications of
pregnancy (premature miscarriages, unexplained fetal death, or premature birth)
and the presence of antiphospholipid antibodies. https://www.mayoclinic.org/
diseases-conditions/antiphospholipid-syndrome/symptoms-causes/syc-20355831.

4. A test made in early pregnancy to detect congenital abnormalities in the fetus.
A tiny tissue sample is taken from the villi of the chorion, which forms the fetal
part of the placenta. https://www.mayoclinic.org/tests-procedures/chorionic-villus-
sampling/.

5. J. A. Dipietro, "Maternal Stress in Pregnancy: Considerations for Fetal
Development," *Journal of Adolescent Health* 51, no. 2 (2012): S3–S8. https://doi.
org/10.1016/j.jadohealth.2012.04.008

6. J. O'Leary, C. Gaziano, and J. Warland, "Gifts from the Deceased Sibling to
Siblings Born After Loss," *International Journal of Prenatal Perinatal Psychology and
Medicine* 23, no. 1/2 (2011): 415–29.

7. Ellen Nelles Leger, RN, PhD, *Tears Change Us: A Spiritual and Stress Management
Guide for Tough Times* (Stressed for Success, Etc., 2015), www.ellenleger.com.

CHAPTER 4

1. https://www.biography.com/people/elizabeth-cady-stanton-9492182.

2. Amniocentesis is a prenatal test in which a small amount of amniotic fluid is
removed from the sac surrounding the fetus for testing. During pregnancy, the
fetus is surrounded by amniotic fluid, a substance much like water. Amniotic fluid
contains live fetal cells and other substances, such as alpha-fetoprotein. These
substances provide important information about your baby's health before birth.

3. A level II ultrasound is similar to a standard ultrasound. The difference is that your doctor will get more detailed information from the level II ultrasound. Your doctor may focus on specific parts of your baby's body, such as his or her brain, heart, or other organs. It can help check your baby for some birth defects, such as Down syndrome (https://www.webmd.com/baby/level-ii-ultrasound).

4. Cervical cerclage, also known as a cervical stitch, is a treatment for cervical insufficiency: when the cervix starts to shorten and open too early during a pregnancy, causing either a late miscarriage or a preterm birth (https://en.wikipedia.org/wiki/Cervical_cerclage).

5. https://starlegacyfoundation.org; https://pregnancyafterlosssupport.org.

6. J. O'Leary and L. Parker, "Parenting Your Baby before Birth," a relaxation experience for parents during pregnancy. Available at https://starlegacyfoundation .org.

CHAPTER 5

1. An anterior placenta is positioned on the front wall of your womb, on your belly side. About a third of moms-to-be have an anterior placenta.

2. https://www.tommys.org/pregnancy-information/im-pregnant/sleep-position-pregnancy-qa, accessed June 22, 2019.

3. A nonstress test (NST), also known as CTG (cardiotocography) or electronic fetal heart rate monitoring, is a common prenatal test used to check on a baby's health. During a nonstress test a baby's heart rate is monitored to see how it responds to the baby's movements.

4. A biophysical profile (BPP) is a prenatal ultrasound evaluation of fetal well-being involving a scoring system, with the score being termed Manning's score. It is often done when an NST is nonreactive or for other obstetrical indications.

5. Robin S. Cronin et al., "An Individual Participant Data Meta-Analysis of Maternal Going-to-Sleep Position, Interactions with Fetal Vulnerability, and the Risk of Late Stillbirth," *EClinicalMedicine* 10 (April 2019): 49–57.

6. J. Warland, J. Dorrian, J. L. Morrison, and L. M. O'Brien, "Maternal Sleep during Pregnancy and Poor Fetal Outcomes: A Scoping Review of the Literature with Meta-Analysis," *Sleep Medicine Reviews* 41 (2018): 197–219.

7. https://www.mindfetalness.com/, accessed June 22, 2019.

CHAPTER 6

1. Thank you to psychologist Rosarii O'Donnell-Connorton from Tipperary, Ireland, for this lovely wording of an "inside baby," a term she uses with her clients.

2. C. Cirulli Lanham, *Pregnancy after a Loss: A Guide to Pregnancy after a Miscarriage, Stillbirth or Infant Death* (New York: Berkley Books, 1999).

3. Christine Nightingale, BA (psychology), Reiki master, certified hypnotist, aromatherapist, spirit baby communicator, nightingalehealing.com.

4. T. Attig, "Relearning the World: Making and Finding Meanings," in *Meaning Reconstruction and the Experience of Loss*, ed. R. Neimeyer (Washington, DC: American Psychological Association, 2001): 33–73.

CHAPTER 7

1. A. E. P. Heazell et al., "Stillbirth Is Associated with Perceived Alterations in Fetal Activity—Findings from an International Case Control Study," *BMC Pregnancy and Childbirth* 17, no 369 (2017). DOI 10.1186/s12884-017-1555-6.

2. https://starlegacyfoundation.org.

3. http://www.hellonorah.com/blog/familyprep.

4. https://www.dona.org/what-is-a-doula/.

5. http://www.calmbirth.org/mp3/calm-birth.

6. A measure of the physical condition of a newborn infant. It is obtained by adding points (2, 1, or 0) for heart rate, respiratory effort, muscle tone, response to stimulation, and skin coloration; a score of 10 represents the best possible condition.

7. https://stillstandingmag.com/2018/11/15/raising-a-rainbow-a-brand-new-layer-of-grief/?utm_sq=g1tebvvnfu&fbclid=IwAR24IPp5nX7UktWNys6vtSBQid-ZuVMwUa-Tej8CQZcDqX4JSbB0H89qL5E.

CHAPTER 8

1. www.bellybelly.com.au/breastfeeding/cluster. The exact reasons why cluster feeding happens are unknown. However, experts assume cluster feeding is a way babies boost breastmilk production during growth spurts. Your baby's stomach grows rapidly during the first few months of life, and your body must produce more milk to meet the increased demand.

2. https://www.ispid.org.

3. https://starlegacyfoundation.org.

CHAPTER 9

1. https://starlegacyfoundation.org/; https://www.sands.org.uk/; https://pillarsofstrength.com.au/.

2. Cathy Blanford, *Something Happened: A Book for Children and Parents Who Have Experienced Pregnancy Loss* (Something Happened Handbook, 2012). Available at https://centering.org/.

CHAPTER 10

1. Phyllis Rolfe Silverman, *Never Too Young to Know: Death in Children's Lives* (New York: Oxford University Press, 2000).

2. E. Hunter, *Sophia Lyons Fahs: A Bibliography* (Boston: Beacon Press, 1966).

3. https://www.zerotothree.org/resources/1073-talking-about-the-loss-of-a-baby-with-young-siblings.

4. https://www.scholastic.com/teachers/articles/teaching-content/ages-stages-how-children-use-magical-thinking/.

5. A rainbow baby is a baby born shortly after the loss of a previous baby due to miscarriage, stillbirth, or death in infancy. This term is given to these special babies because a rainbow typically follows a storm, giving us hope of what's to come.

6. https://gesellinstitute.org/.

7. J. Warland, J. O'Leary, and H. McCutcheon, "Born after Infant Loss: The Experiences of Subsequent Children," *Midwifery* 27, no. 5 (2011): 628–33.

8. J. O'Leary, C. Gaziano, and J. Warland, "Gifts from the Deceased Sibling to Siblings Born after Loss," *International Journal of Prenatal Perinatal Psychology and Medicine* 23, no. 1/2 (2011): 415–29.

9. J. O'Leary, C. Gaziano, and C. Thorwick, "Born after Loss: The Invisible Child in Adulthood," *Journal of Pre and Perinatal Psychology and Health* 21, no. 1 (2006): 3–23.

CHAPTER 12

1. www.goodreads.com/quotes/4202-what-we-once.

2. Hyaline membrane disease is a condition in newborn babies in which the lungs are deficient in surfactant, preventing their proper expansion and causing the formation of hyaline material in the lung spaces.

3. P. Rosenblatt, "Protective Parenting after the Death of a Child," *Journal of Personal and Interpersonal Loss* 5, no. 4 (2000): 343–60.

4. https://www.facebook.com/events/october-15th-wave-of-light.../249211161944550/.

5. Mollybears.org.

6. P. Keech, *Mothering an Angel* (Edina, MN: Beavers Pond Press, 2001).

7. K. Haugan, *Journey* (St. Cloud, MN: Sunray Publishing, 2007).

CHAPTER 13

1. Cathy Blanford, *Something Happened: A Book for Children and Parents Who Have Experienced Pregnancy Loss* (Something Happened Handbook, 2012).

2. https://starlegacyfoundation.org/.

Index

About the Authors

Joann O'Leary has a PhD and MPH from the University of Minnesota, as well as an MS in psychology from Queen's University Belfast, Northern Ireland, and is endorsed as a level IV in infant mental health. She has a background in preschool special education and eighteen years in clinical practice as a parent-infant specialist in a high-risk perinatal center, where she worked individually with families and facilitated pregnancy-after-loss support groups. She has published a book, two book chapters, and two video productions on the pregnancy that follows loss. She was a 2016 Fulbright Specialist at University College Cork, Ireland, and is now a consultant to Star Legacy Foundation facilitating pregnancy-after-loss support groups. Her research and clinical focus is how perinatal loss and the pregnancy that follows impact parents, children, and extended family members.

Lynnda Parker is a registered nurse and holds degrees in education and nursing along with attending graduate studies in nurse midwifery. She has worked for twenty-five years in high-risk perinatal nursing. She founded the Pregnancy After Loss Support Groups with Dr. O'Leary, where they cofacilitated the groups. She also taught childbirth preparation classes specially designed for pregnancy after loss. She developed a pregnancy class, "Bodyworks," for women experiencing a complicated pregnancy. She has assisted Dr. O'Leary with research, and together they have provided professional education for physicians, midwives, nurses, social workers, chaplains, and educators. She is currently an adjunct instructor in nursing.

Dr. Margaret M. Murphy is a registered midwife and registered general nurse with over twenty years of clinical midwifery experience. Her research area is pregnancy after loss. She has been a faculty member at the School of Nursing and Midwifery, University College Cork, Ireland, and is a member of the Pregnancy Loss Research Group, INFANT Research Centre, Cork, Ireland. She delivers bereavement education courses to undergraduate and postgraduate students and is lead author of "Irish Standards for Perinatal Bereavement Education," two book chapters, and over thirty publications. She is the treasurer and executive board member of International Stillbirth Alliance.

Dr. Jane Warland is a midwife and faculty member at the University of South Australia. Since suffering the unexplained full-term stillbirth of her daughter Emma in 1993, she has been a passionate researcher of preventative and modifiable risk factors for stillbirth as well as a strong advocate for promoting public and maternity care provider awareness of stillbirth. Jane practiced as a nurse-midwife for thirty years before commencing work as an academic in 2008 and has more than one hundred publications, including a book titled *Pregnancy after Loss*, which she wrote and published with her husband, Mike, in 1996.

CPSIA information can be obtained
at www.ICGtesting.com
Printed in the USA
BVHW072049051120
592469BV00002B/3